Implementing Change
in the NHS

Health Services Management Series

Series editor
Stuart Haywood

Health care has become a major issue for western governments. It commands a significant proportion of national wealth, and rising professional and public expectations threaten to increase it yet further. There is a seemingly insatiable demand for additional resources, usually in excess of the general rise in prosperity. Consequently, cost containment has been much in vogue in recent years, finding expression in such policies as priority for lower cost primary medical care.

In the British National Health Service, as in many other countries, market disciplines are largely muted or absent. There are few competitive pressures and thereby incentive for health authorities, hospitals, clinics or professionals to promote efficiency. The alternative in the NHS has been cash-limited financial allocations to health authorities and, more recently, government insistence on cash-releasing 'cost-improvements'.

There has also been increasing attention to NHS management. It is seen as a much more important factor in performance than was the case in the early years of the service. Administrators, for example, were seen mainly as supportive, ensuring systems ran smoothly for professionals who led the development of the service. The idea of managers as a much more positive force responsible for planning and directing development only began to take root in the 1970s, culminating in the appointment of general managers in 1984–6.

Expectations of managers will continue to accelerate, given their higher profile in the organization. The management of NHS resources will become even more challenging since the gap between what is affordable (under any system) and professional and public aspirations is likely to continue to grow. Pressures to improve efficiency will intensify, along with those to ensure that services are more sensitive to the wishes of consumers. Managers will also have to be more rigorous in their examination of the benefits of developments, particularly those utilizing expensive technology.

The rapid development of the role of NHS managers has outstripped the capacity of training institutions and schools of management to respond to their needs. There are relatively few texts which relate management theories and skills to the circumstances of publicly-provided health care. The answer is not to be found in an uncritical transfer of private-sector techniques. A good example is the relative failure of the first four 'demonstration' projects, seeking to introduce clinical management budgeting for acute services.

This series of books is intended to make good a little of the deficiency in suitable educational and training materials, necessary to underpin the development of management. The aim will be to relate advances in theories, systems, techniques and skills to the management of health care organizations, particularly the NHS. The books will be primarily concerned with practical problems and issues of concern to those involved in the management, not just managers.

Implementing Change in the NHS

A guide for general managers

PETER SPURGEON

Director, Health Service Management Centre,
University of Birmingham

and

FREDERICK BARWELL

Consultant Psychologist and Honorary Research Fellow,
Health Service Management Centre,
University of Birmingham

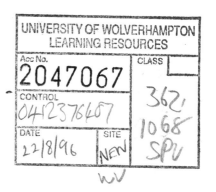
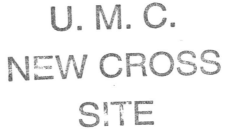

CHAPMAN & HALL
London · New York · Tokyo · Melbourne · Madras

In association with
Health Services Management Centre

UK	Chapman & Hall, 2-6 Boundary Row, London SE1 8HN
USA	Chapman & Hall, 29 West 35th Street, New York NY10001
JAPAN	Chapman & Hall Japan, Thomson Publishing Japan, Hirakawacho Nemoto Building, 7F, 1-7-11 Hirakawa-cho, Chiyoda-ku, Tokyo 102
AUSTRALIA	Chapman & Hall Australia, Thomas Nelson Australia, 102 Dodds Street, South Melbourne, Victoria 3205
INDIA	Chapman & Hall India, R. Seshadri, 32 Second Main Road, CIT East, Madras 600 035

First edition 1991

© 1991 Peter Spurgeon and Frederick Barwell

Typeset in 9½/11 Plantin by Mews Photosetting, Beckenham, Kent

Printed in Great Britain by Page Bros (Norwich) Ltd

ISBN 0 412 37640 7

British Library Cataloguing in Publication Data

Spurgeon, Peter
  Implementing change in the NHS : A guide for
  general managers. - (Health services management series).
  1. Great Britain. National health services. Management
  I. Title II. Barwell, Frederick III. Health Service
  Management Centre IV. Series
  362.1068

ISBN 0-412-37640-7

Library of Congress Cataloging in Publication Data

Spurgeon, P. (Peter)
  Implementing change in the NHS : a guide for general
  managers / Peter Spurgeon and Frederick Barwell. — 1st ed.
      p. cm. — (Health services management series)
  Published in association with Health Services Management Centre.
  Includes bibliographical references (p.) and index.
  ISBN 0-412-37640-7
  1. National Health Service (Great Britain)—Administration.
  2. Health services administration—Great Britain. I. Barwell,
  Frederick, 1952- . II. University of Birmingham. Health Services
  Management Centre. III. Title.
  RA395.G6S68 1991
  362.1'0941—dc20   90-15025
                                                              CIP

Contents

Series editor's preface

The advent of general management in the National Health Service (NHS) has set off a train of seemingly never-ending changes. An internal market for health care, characterized by contracting and competition has followed quickly on the heels of performance related pay, performance review, resource management and efficiency initiatives. All are part of the same initiative which has a momentum of its own.

One effect has been the growing realization that change, in its many manifestations, is ever present and continuous. The days of the 'steady state' – if they ever existed – have gone.

The realization of the new reality is a first step in preparing for it. The next step is to enhance our (already considerable) ability to promote and handle it competently. This book is a contribution to this process.

It updates and deepens understanding of change and suggests practical ways in which they can be managed in the NHS. The authors rightly argue that many other texts do one or the other rather than both. Yet both are essential for a greater competency, something the book's review of the impact of general management suggests is still very necessary.

Stuart Haywood

CHAPTER 1
The emerging culture of the NHS

Introduction

Views held of the National Health Service are increasingly ambivalent if not approaching schizophrenic. The NHS is a major consumer of resources and also the nation's largest single employer. It is still the most popular major institution and many cherish the values enshrined in its inception. Champions of the NHS see the continuing provision of free and equal health care on demand as the defining virtue of the NHS. They are bolstered in this belief by the esteem in which the NHS is held in many other countries and by the numerous countries who have seen the NHS as a model for their own health services.

However, there exists an equally prevalent and contradictory set of views that the NHS is in crisis and toppling on the verge of terminal decay. Critics point to factors such as the constant struggle to reduce waiting lists and lengthy waiting times within a hospital visit. Further problems in supplying the necessary level of potentially life-saving procedures such as dialysis and transplants, together with the much publicized closure of hospital wards has resulted in the view that the NHS is an inefficient and wasteful bureaucracy. The present government's own internal review of the NHS has further fuelled this notion of breakdown and inefficiency.

Morale of NHS staff is accordingly extremely labile. It is sustained for some by a real sense of vocation and for others from the satisfaction of having helped to provide vital care to those in need. Understandably, this morale plummets in the face of financial cutbacks, of long hours and highly critical public attention. It is hardly surprising that with this level of discord the NHS should be subject to scrutiny, and this was indeed exactly what happened with the Management Inquiry in 1983 (Griffiths Report).

The focus of this text is upon the post-Griffiths phase, and in particular it examines how managers have tackled the implications of the Report. The aim of our approach is to understand better the processes involved and also to help managers evaluate their own contribution to the change process and as a consequence to maximize their effectiveness.

Evolution or change?

It was interesting to observe reaction within the service during the initial phases of implementing the Griffiths proposals. There were broadly three main categories of individual response.

1. A positive desire to grasp the opportunities offered by general management; this appeared a straightforward reaction but was typically associated with varying degrees of haziness about quite what would be involved.
2. A sense of frustration born out of a belief that the NHS was constantly being reorganized (previously there had been significant reorganizations in 1974 and 1982) and a feeling that if left alone the system would 'settle down' and improve; there may be a clue here to the prevailing NHS culture about change since the frequency of change contrasts sharply with many private sector organizations where much more frequent changes are instituted in accord with a rapidly changing market.
3. A rather world-weary and cynical view of yet another new idea which given time, and if we all just sit tight, will probably disappear like all the rest.

A rich source of knowledge in understanding the process of change could be tapped if we knew where individuals holding these views currently stand. This idea will be developed throughout the book as it is a basic tenet of our approach that understanding the way in which individuals perceive change is vital to managing the process.

Each of the individual viewpoints expressed above assumes that general management is a discontinuous, almost revolutionary change. However, at the institutional level the advent of general management can be credibly described as part of an evolutionary series of developments. Mounting criticism of the NHS in the 1960s pointed to the organization's inability to adapt sufficiently quickly to the changing needs of the population. The comments contained in the Griffiths Report clearly echo these earlier concerns. The outcome was of course the first reorganization in 1974. Perhaps the most important facets of this reorganization were

1. The creation of Regions and Areas as executive authorities
2. The introduction of teams of managers at District, Area and Regional levels charged with pursuing consensus management decisions
3. The creation of Community Health Councils to represent consumer interests at District level; and
4. A new planning system.

Whatever the merits of the advocated structures they were rapidly constrained by economic pressures, and 1976 saw the introduction of the concept of cash limits. The election in 1979 of a Conservative government with a commitment to reducing public spending served to intensify this pattern of tighter control of costs in areas such as health. Preliminary initiatives included the Rayner Scrutinies and Regional Reviews culminating with the second reorganization in 1982. This was essentially a simplifying and streamlining process with the abolition of Area authorities and a reduction in the number of consultative professional bodies. It also heralded a more centralized structure emphasizing greater accountability to managers.

In retrospect it is not difficult to discern the consistent pattern of economic and political pressures which inexorably led to the setting up of the NHS Management Inquiry in 1983. Under the chairmanship of Sir Roy Griffiths, the brief given to the inquiry team was to 'review initiatives to improve the efficiency of the health service and to advise on the management action needed to secure the best value for money and the best possible service to patients'. This brief was very much in keeping with the chain of prior events.

Although the evolutionists have justifiably argued that the Inquiry was simply a further step along a developmental path, the impact of resultant recommendations represents a major change in approach to health service management. In our view the scale of these changes is extremely far reaching. The basic contention of this text is that introduction of general management to the NHS is a fundamental and probably irreversible change in the way health care is provided. This theme will be developed in subsequent chapters as the work of managers in handling the change process is explored.

Griffiths: recommendations and reactions

The focus of the Griffiths inquiry team was on management systems rather than on specific problems such as costs or manpower. In attempting to report quickly, the team chose to make recommendations within the scope of existing legislation and also to make use of previous initiatives of the 1970s. They highlighted the lack of a clearly defined management function and in particular the absence of individual responsibility. Although acknowledging the merits of consensus management they felt it was too slow and cumbersome resulting in delay in the management process.

The recommendations of the inquiry team have been the subject of much commentary. The key elements are presented here as the backcloth to much of the change that is examined later. Briefly, the Griffiths Report recommended

1. The establishment of a National Health Service Management Board to provide a central management function
2. The creation of a general management function throughout all levels of the service with individual general managers being appointed at District and Unit level who are accountable for the service provided. It was noted that these managers should be drawn from any discipline within the NHS or indeed from managers outside the service
3. That as far as possible day-to-day management decisions should be devolved to the unit of operation
4 That the service should seek to involve clinicians more closely in the management process
5. The service should endeavour to be more aware and more sensitive to the needs of the consumer
6. The management structures within each District should have greater flexibility and attempt to incorporate the varying patterns of needs within different populations.

Associated with these essential recommendations were proposals about cost improvement programmes and management budgets to bring about a more effective relationship between inputs, workload and service objectives.

This relatively brief report contained within it the impetus to major change to practice and procedures in health care management. Essentially it sought to move the NHS from what was largely a passively administered service to one that was actively managed. A transition such as this may appear deceptively simple, and initially some health authorities appeared to equate the implementation of general management merely as the appointment of the designated managers and a few rather cosmetic overtures to the recommendations of the report. It is probably now widely accepted that this superficial approach was not adequate and that, in truth, the adoption of general management in the NHS required a significant shift in practices for all professional groups together with a reassessment of service priorities.

The brevity of the Griffiths report misled many as to its level of implication and unfortunately seemed to carry an almost inherent potential for misunderstanding. This confusion seemed partly to be due to the fact that if initiatives are not spelt out in precise detail then for some individuals they remain unclear. This problem was exacerbated by the report's relatively high level of conceptual analysis which introduced scope for different interpretations.

Scepticism was certainly present within the NHS about the merits of the Griffiths proposals. There was indeed some justification to the belief that the very short timescale of the inquiry had led to an over-simplistic, and perhaps naïve, assumption that the model of private sector profit orientation so enthusiastically endorsed by the government would simply generalize to the NHS. It was quite widely held that the inquiry team had failed to grasp many of the complexities of the health care sector. As the implementation of the proposals has proceeded there is increasing support for this view as various subtle issues about managing the provision of health care emerge. Two excellent retrospective articles by Klein (1985) and by Allen and Lupton (1988) point in particular to the failure to recognize fully the complexities of both the political context and management systems within the NHS.

Klein argues that it is the publicly financed nature of health care plus the view that managers are concerned with containing the 'cost explosion' that 'help to identify why management in health care is peculiarly difficult, as well as different from management in other spheres'. In the private sector the goal of maximizing profit and market share is of paramount importance although there may be on occasions special reasons for departing from this goal. In contrast in health care the achievement of increased activity (and notionally therefore market share) often results in increasing costs (and public cost primarily).

Additionally, the 'product' in health care is rather different in nature from that of other goods on the market (Abel-Smith 1976). The patient is not likely to read consumer surveys of the best hernia or heart surgeons or be able to shop around prior to use. Thus the provider–consumer relationship in health care is not like that of other goods.

Similarly the manager in health care must maintain some sort of balance between promoting innovation and stifling development. Again the private sector would find this situation more readily reconcilable as the market would determine whether proposed innovations were pursued or shelved. Furthermore, the goals and aspirations of clinicians and other professional staff within the NHS may be directly at odds with the managers' requirement to meet external political and financial pressures. These points serve to illustrate the complex area in which managers in health care must operate.

In terms of management systems Allen and Lupton (1988) have utilized contingency theory to point out that no single formula will solve the management needs of all organizations. The nature of each organization is sufficiently different to demand an individual management style. This evidence, they argue, is in complete contrast to the assumption behind the implementation of general management in the NHS. They point both to the political and financial environment in which the NHS functions and highlight a clash between the inherent organizational values of caring for the sick and vulnerable with the economic market place orientation.

The current explorations of internal markets and of expanding private health care funding represent attempts to resolve some of these competing pressures. The degree to which 'provider units' create real competition and choice for the consumer will provide the crucial test of the applicability of market forces to health care.

Structure of the book

The misgivings and arguments presented above are important and must be borne in mind. Nonetheless, general management is in place in the NHS and is probably here to stay for the foreseeable future. General management represents a radical cultural challenge to existing work practices and therefore is part of both structural and process changes within the organization. A fundamental assumption of the approach adopted here is that general management in the NHS is synonymous with managing organizational change and innovation.

Understanding how managers bring about change cannot be fully tackled by research which merely concentrates on what managers do in the course of their jobs. For too long management research has simply collected descriptive data on what activities supposedly 'effective' managers carry out. This has resulted in either a wide-ranging diversity of activities, confirming only that good managers do things in different ways, or a few summarized common characteristics so general as to be of little theoretical or practical value. Prior to initiating any action a manager has a view or perspective on the organization, which comprises both how the organization 'looks' at present and in a dynamic sense how he/she would like it to 'look' in the future. This latter perception is vital because it clarifies the changes that need to take place in order to create the organization required. This perception of the future organization and the deficit between 'how it is' and 'how it will be' is what determines managerial behaviour. This view is clearly expressed by Weick (1979) who sees organizations not in structural or functional terms but as reflecting the thought processes of the individuals and collectives who comprise the organization. In order to understand the process of change we must know how the change agent views the process of change and the goals, values and expectations on which this process is founded.

The rest of the book is divided into several distinct sections and it may help the reader to understand the thinking behind the structure.

Chapters 2, 3 and 4 provide a theoretical backcloth examining initially the nature and role of general management, both inside and outside the NHS. Chapter 4 provides an overview of the various theories and models that attempt to interpret the process of organizational change.

Chapters 5, 6 and 7 provide a practical perspective for managers on how individual managers view and attempt to bring about change. Case study material is utilized to demonstrate the initial importance of managers' mental models of change and instruments and techniques are suggested as to how managers might examine and improve the effectiveness of their own approach to change.

The authors conducted a research programme to capture the early activities of general managers in their attempts to implement organizational innovations. This research and the measures used are described in Chapters 8 and 9.

Finally, in Chapter 10 an overview is given as to how the findings and model developed in the text can be integrated with the ever-increasing number of proposed changes in the workings of the National Health Service, in particular how the radical propositions contained within the White Paper 'Working for patients' need to be incorporated into a mental picture of a new health-care system.

CHAPTER 2
The nature of general management

Barriers to change

We have seen that the Griffiths inquiry had suggested a number of managerial deficiences which, in its view, lay at the heart of a range of inefficiencies within the health service. It is not hard to understand why such a focused report might provoke at least a slightly defensive reaction, particularly from administrators. It would be unfair to describe the prevailing attitude as one of resistance, but implementing the inquiry team's recommendations was seen at best as a challenge and at worst as a formidable task.

Efforts to secure the level of change implied by general management are inevitably likely to encounter a form of institutional inertia. Specifically, the NHS contained within it a series of established patterns and practice which were always going to make radical change difficult.

The NHS has a very strong tradition of 'professionalism'; so much so that the term 'tribalism' has been used to capture the strength of identity within the various groups. As a consequence of this occupational kinship professional concerns have come to dominate more general managerial issues. It is perhaps not surprising, given the personal nature of the services provided, that professional codes should be a dominant concern. Nonetheless, other industries flourish where high levels of professional competence are demanded and where management co-exists as a far stronger faction. It was recognized that a key component of general management in the NHS had to be the creation of a superordinate level of management above and beyond professional groupings with a legitimate role to manage resources for the provision of service goals.

A serious consequence of the ongoing strength of occupational group identity was that the NHS had come to represent a plurality of views and priorities as to what the organization should be doing. This is highlighted and exemplified by the role of the medical profession. Clinicians are, and should be, the main allocators of NHS resources, although few have any direct involvement in management, or even a clear understanding of how their decisions affect the management of the service.

Harrison (1988) has recently examined the impact of general management upon staff groups, in particular upon the medical profession and nurses. He suggests that there is an inherent logical contradiction between notions of professionalism and notions of management, since professionalism is primarily concerned with the application of independent judgement. However, he also considers that conflict will occur only if the two groups wish to pursue different objectives. This may explain why much predicted conflict often fails to materialize. Certainly, the BMA's initial response to Griffiths was hostile, essentially characterizing it as an attack upon clinical freedom. However, most of the recent initiatives such as the introduction of resource management or performance indicators are being couched in terms of increased rationality of decision-making and have not produced widescale confrontation. Perhaps managers are wisely attempting to get such systems in place before utilizing their potential to control clinical behaviour. Alternatively, it may be that general managers have not as yet fully grasped the nettle of clinical control and the real challenges to the medical profession may still come from outside the service in the form of further cash limits or constraints upon professional groups.

In the nursing profession the reaction to Griffiths was even more hostile. This hostility was fuelled by fears of loss of status and anxieties about the potential control of nurses by non-nurses. It is evident that many senior nurse managers have fared badly in the appointment of general managers and the associated reshuffling of responsibilities. However, there has been a compensatory development in terms of emphasis on quality of care and many nurses have been given key responsibilities in this area. The long term effects are probably still equivocal and will again be much influenced by external factors such as level of pay and retention conditions.

It is worth noting that in the two example groups cited above there is a clear and powerful external influence upon the service which may be the key to many initiatives. There are echoes here of the discussion in Chapter 1 of the public context in which NHS managers function. An especially important consequence of this is that for many people general management is synonymous with financial cuts and the inevitable correlate of reductions in service.

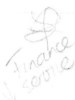

Clearly this belief may have very negative implications for the acceptability of the general management ethos. The arrival of general managers at a time when financial support to the service is being restricted should not be treated as one and the same issue. Finally, a considerable barrier to introducing general management in the NHS is that there is a widespread lack of clarity about just what is involved in general management. The movement from passive maintenance of the institution to a proactive management stance may well release valuable managerial energy but equally it is vital that this force should be clear about what its objectives are and how to achieve them. In the early days, rather than addressing these problems the service became over-concerned, sometimes to the point of obsession, with who was going to be appointed as the general manager in their district or unit. We will examine this aspect in some detail in Chapter 3. However, it is initially worthwhile to look at the manner of the NHS response to understanding general management.

Attempts to define general management in the NHS

The National Health Service Training Authority (NHSTA), recognizing the lack of clear vision of general management or a proven formula which could be imported from elsewhere, commissioned a paper to spell out the implications of general management in the NHS. This paper, prepared by Gordon Best (1984) emphasized the issue of 'making desirable change happen'. Specifically, the paper highlighted the need for clearly stating objectives to provide direction and to facilitate the assessment of achievement. In summary it states that 'general management can be seen to consist of the development, utilization and periodic revision of a number of interdependent, mutually reinforcing strategies which relate what is desirable to what is possible in order to make desired change happen'.

Additionally Best also recognized that the scale and diversity of the change required was enormous and that it would be unreasonable to expect such an upheaval to be achieved in less than five to ten years. Quite correctly much of the argument within the document was concerned to show the need for more strategic thinking by managers in a number of spheres. However, in retrospect the paper may have contained a stylistic error in that it offered an illustrative management structure as a visible target for immediate progress.

It may be coincidence but much of the early efforts of general managers were devoted to devising new management structures. Although a necessary process, it is also true that the NHS as an organization has tended, to its disadvantage, to equate structure change with the process of change.

Change is an elusive concept and it is often helpful to make explicit those aspects where change is being sought. There are many potential levels of change.

1. The overall goals and objectives of the NHS as an institution
2. The policies and programmes operating within the service
3. Specific outcomes in terms of health care delivery
4. Managerial procedures, systems and structures
5. Behaviour and attitudes of the managers.

Clearly, there will be an interaction between these as one initiative flows into another, although the NHS has typically tended to expect change to follow from policy statements, structural reorganizations and new procedures and systems. Our analysis of the change process in Chapter 4 suggests that if general management is to succeed then managers will have to dramatically broaden their emphasis to include all of the other elements listed above.

A clear vision of organizational goals and objectives, incorporating outcome measures, is essential. Alongside this must come the relatively new and challenging issue of changing attitudes and behaviour. In many respects the argument presented here serves to underline the need for individual managers to move in a consistent manner from their personal vision of the organization to their own behaviour as an agent of this change process.

It is not our intention here to record in any detail specific events that have taken place as a result of general management. However, a brief look at some initiatives will give an indication of the approach to change and why, we shall argue, a more individual cognitive map of the change process is essential for success.

General management at work in the NHS

It is interesting to note that David Bowden in his presidential address to the

Institute of Health Service Management, 1988, said that 'there is no doubt that the introduction of general management into the National Health Service has become a signficant success story'. Of particular importance in reaching this conclusion was his view that there had been a shift from managers being judged by success with managing the processes of the organization to being judged on results. There is a comfortable assurance that this sort of movement must be right. It makes sense for managers to be judged on what they achieve. However, this is a rather more subtle and complex shift than it appears at first. The real change is the inclusion of outcome into the evaluation of managerial performance. Previously it had been a case of emphasizing process to such an extent that outcome was almost ignored. It would be equally inappropriate to make a similar form of unbalanced emphasis in the new circumstances. Managing the process is still equally important, for without the supportive infra-structure that results from process orientation then desired outcomes are unlikely to be achieved. Flanagan and Spurgeon (1987) have shown that NHS managers are judged to be effective largely by how well they handle the various process issues. Indeed Bowden goes on to argue that equally critical to successful management are considerations such as good public relations, demonstrating respect and value for one's staff and providing leadership through direction, openness and support. All these might once upon a time have been thought of as process variables.

Further support for not divorcing process from results is to be found in the work of Smith (1987) who collected self-perceptions from over 50 unit general managers on the emphasis of their activities during their first year in the post. Just as examples, the first three listed activities were

1. Managing change, involving open meetings to explain the new systems; trying to break down some of the established professional barriers; and coping with the anxieties and tension of change within the departments
2. Developing relations with others including District General Manager, other UGMs and the authority members
3. Building a network of contacts through which the organization might be influenced.

All these are essential tasks to the achievement of effective general management as judged by output but they are in themselves process orientated.

Perhaps the most systematic study to date of the introduction of general management into the health service is described in the Templeton Series of reports. The study team led by Rosemary Stewart described various facets of the role of the DGM and these have been published in a series of 'issue studies' by the NHSTA. In addition Williams and Dopson (1988), members of the research team, have written a summary paper relating some of the findings to more theoretical models.

The project took the form of a longitudinal 'tracer' study of how a sample of twenty DGMs tackled their jobs during the first two years of their appointments. The immediate aims of the study were to describe the issues encountered during this period, how they set about tackling these problems and the nature of differences in approach. The sample of DGMs was not truly representative but included a range of District sizes, and a range of prior backgrounds within the DGMs themselves. As Williams and Dopson pointed out this method inevitably resulted in a restricted perception of relevant issues but it did allow in-depth analysis of a rapidly changing number of situations. Some of the particular issues discussed illustrate the early face of general management in the NHS.

The Templeton Series (No. 5) which discusses the involvement of doctors in management is a good example of many of the tensions and problems encountered in the introduction of general management. We have previously mentioned the rather suspicious attitude of the medical profession at large to the new management initiatives. At an individual level many doctors feared an attack on clinical freedom and medical autonomy. In particular they feared the 'commercial' weighting of decisions, believing that there would be a finance-led view of health care which would force doctors to practice upon economic rather than clinical criteria.

Similarly, managers saw doctors as fundamentally constraining their options by entering into clinical activity without concern for the cost or for the wider resource implications. Often it is also difficult for managers to enter fully into a positive debate about such issues since their lack of clinical expertise makes them vulnerable to technical and professional detail. At the same time there has been little incentive for doctors to involve themselves in management. To do so would mean that not only do they depart from a very competitive career route but they may also suffer financial loss and possible conflict with medical colleagues.

There is here a reflection of quite different values and cultural norms. Rarely do doctors receive any training or education in management. Their entire professional socialization is orientated to making them confident and independent decision makers putting patient need above all other considerations. In contrast, managers are trained to look for broad organizational perspectives and to be aware of the interactions and interdependencies of different work groups.

As the Templeton reports make clear there is a great danger of stereotyping with such views. However, a wide range of views was present within the sample, ranging from one DGM who sought directly to control the excessive power of doctors to other more moderate managers who were trying to find ways of utilizing medical skills in the management process. A number of strategies for achieving this involvement were identified.

1. Reorganizing individual contributions and building on these to tackle particular problems within their own medical specialities
2. Recognizing the ability of some doctors in management skills which are often frequently practised but not always appreciated
3. Developing doctors' management ability through special seminars and projects
4. Demonstrating the value of general management by helping to solve some outstanding problem or long-term issues and hence encouraging reciprocal support and involvement.

It was revealing that several of the sample repeatedly stressed the key issue of doctors in management and yet approached it 'diffidently and in a piecemeal fashion'. In some instances this has resulted in many battles over isssues which, if a fully developed strategy had existed, might not even have been worth fighting over.

Beckhard (1985) outlines the following key features of planning for change.

1. Developing with the key people a clear vision of the desired future
2. Understanding and evaluating the current situation
3. Planning on overall strategy for change
4. Working towards short-term interim objectives within the strategy.

These elements are very much akin to the approach we advocate here which focuses upon the critical process of managers developing an individual cognitive model of the change process incorporating a realistic picture of the current situation, a vision of the desired future and an awareness of actions that will create this desired transition. It is worth emphasizing that a single 'best approach' is not appropriate. Rather the key to successful change is that each manager must evolve a cognitive map which is consistent at each point. Later chapters will discuss ways in which this map may be described and how it can be utilized to guide the management of change.

Individual interpretation of vision and process is a point made by Williams and Dopson (*op. cit*) in concluding that 'there is no single homogeneous general management culture'. DGMs differ in their interpretation of the role, in their attitudes and in their actions. Once again the vision, objectives and actions of an integrated cognitive model are highlighted in any attempt to understand the success of managers in bringing about change. Many similar examples may be found in the ways in which DGMs saw and introduced District Management Boards. Apart from the differences in sizes of the Boards or the value of individuals on the Board there were also clear differences in the perceived primary function which reflected the way in which the DGMs saw their role in general management. Some Boards were advisory, others had strong corporate executive responsibilities, some were fostered as collectives for breeding a shared culture whilst yet others were more like battlegrounds where issues could be thrashed out and resolved. There were similar diverse patterns to be observed in the relationships of DGMs and UGMs and also in the pattern of devolved power to unit level. Such differences are in no sense regrettable, for it is entirely appropriate that the ideas and preferences of chief executives (DGMs) should influence their organization's response to general management. It is of course the paramount challenge for general managers to ensure that all other members of the organization share this vision and behave in ways consistent with the achievement of these goals. It will be interesting to see if similar variations occur in the construction of health boards in terms of the recommendations for executive and non-executive directors.

Recently there has been a much greater sense of local control in health authorities and a relatively new acceptance of the need to emphasize learning and development amongst managers. Apart from these important areas he supports the view that it is the sense of change that is most exciting. He describes an organizational culture of initiative, urgency and vitality as the revolution that is taking place. Just how far down this road the current NHS can be said to have travelled is debatable. However, it is certainly in accord with our earlier contention that the advent of general management is not a gradual evolution but a radical and major cultural adjustment. The degree of change is really very considerable involving senior managers in understanding their new role but also communicating the new culture to the rest of the organization. Our research programme was oriented towards examining how they are approaching this task, and from this identifying some of the features key to success.

However, before we look at the change process and the response of general managers in the health service it will be useful to ensure that we have a clear picture of general management as a whole. To this end we will consider the nature of general management outside the NHS.

General management in a wider context

The study of management is a relatively new phenomenon in social science. Compared to major analyses of the functioning of organizations from a bureaucratic or economic perspective the focus on management is very much a child of the twentieth century. Modern systems of thinking as exemplified by Kast and Rosenzweig (1985) illustrate the struggle of management to emerge as a distinct discipline.

They suggest four initial sub-systems.

1. **Goals and values sub-system** – culture, philosophy and overall goals
2. **Technical sub-system** – knowledge, techniques, facilities, equipment
3. **Psychological sub-system** – attitudes, perceptions, motivation, communication, interpersonal relations
4. **Structural sub-system** – tasks, work flow, information flow, procedure, rules.

Superimposed upon these is the **managerial sub-system** composed of the standard managerial tasks of goal setting, planning, assembling resources, organizing, implementing and controlling. The difficulty for management is that it spans all the other processes, and furthermore once they are all functioning effectively management is virtually indistinguishable from them. It is precisely because of this lack of a clearly separated identity that management is often denigrated by other groups with questions such as 'what do they do?' and 'what would happen if they weren't here? The likelihood is that in the very short term the organization would continue to function but as decisions go unmade and activities remain unplanned and lacking in co-ordination so the organization would begin to disintegrate. Of course others could take over these functions but then they become the managers. Another repercussion is that it is really only relatively recently that management is beginning to acquire the status of a profession in its own right. Despite these concerns there have been a number of academic enquiries into the nature of general managerial activity.

If we consider the general manager as someone with the ultimate responsibility for the running of an organization we have in a rather simplistic way captured the essential ingredients of general management. Many definitions have been proferred although one that particularly appeals, because of its emphasis upon holistic aspects, is offered by Andrews (1980) 'Management may be defined as the direction of informed, efficient, planned and purposeful conduct of complex organized activity. Its diverse forms in all kinds of businesses always include the integration of the work of functional managers or specialists.'

A recent text by Aguilar (1988) draws upon a number of case studies and leads to a description of the tasks and roles of general management which would find much sympathy elsewhere, although there is a particularly strong emphasis on strategic direction. The first two task areas Aguilar identifies involve creating and maintaining organizational values and setting strategic objectives and direction. Both areas have received considerable emphasis within the Health Service as the impact of general management has unfolded. The values and norms of an organization influence how its staff will operate. The nature of this value-driven philosophy can be very varied, perhaps being innovative or risk orientated, perhaps very professional and 'up-market'. The key point is that the general managerial function should be critical to the establishment and diffusion of these values. Clearly, the quality of care initiative in the NHS will only be effective if all staff are imbued with appropriate values and beliefs about how they interact with patients. Many individuals who have been given responsibility for quality assurance in their Districts may struggle unless they can encourage their DGMs and UGMs to show personal and organizational commitment to these goals.

A critical input to the establishment of persuasive organizational values is the development of clear strategic goals and a shared sense of direction. The general manager must understand the capabilities of his organization, the environment in which it operates and be capable of articulating policies and plans that integrate and optimize these features. Strategic analysis in a complex setting is not easy and many good operational managers find the transition to such strategic thinking difficult to achieve. Some managers feel more at ease with the familiar and routine, others are unable or unwilling to create the necessary time and distance from day-to-day events to assess the strategic direction of an organization. Interestingly, in Health Authorities, the development of information support systems has been hampered by a lack of clarity of goals and objectives. Both the roles identified here are critical to organizational success and, as shall be demonstrated later, fundamental to the process of organizational change.

Despite the emphasis given to strategic action Aguilar also recognizes that the general manager is not divorced from more immediate operational matters. He/she is ultimately responsible for the allocation of resources of all kinds, for the organization of work and motivation of staff and probably for trouble shooting and decision making about contingencies. Undoubtedly there will be many other support staff involved and the degree of involvement may vary but the ultimate responsibility lies at this level.

In assessing the impact of these various managerial tasks Aguilar concludes that there are four key roles which the general manager must play.

1. **Instigator**. Basically this involves the general manager in supplying the push or momentum to ensure that change, projects and plans come to fruition. It may involve overcoming resistance but equally may need to incorporate the acceptance of failure.
2. **Priority setter**. It is often difficult to discern whether some tasks and goals have a lower priority than others, especially for staff in the middle of the organization who perhaps have responsibility only for short or medium term goals. It is up to the general manager to determine from his strategic

analysis which of the organization's goals should have priority and then to ensure that these are implemented.

3. **Integrator.** In large organizations the diversity of activities can sometimes make it difficult to see how individual patterns of activity fit with the whole. The general manager is in a position to see them in their entirety and then produce a sense of cohesion and integration.

4. **Taskmaster.** The essence of this role is to avoid complacency. The general manager must in a whole manner of ways (rewards, feedback, etc.) seek to promote continued improvement in performance.

The earlier study of general managers by Kotter (1982) resulted in a similar set of descriptors. (Roles are of course expressed in different terms and this variation in language used to describe managers in different studies is a topic to which we shall return.) The approach of Kotter's study was to examine in some detail the work patterns of just fifteen general managers in a range of industrial contexts. Despite this very individualized approach he identified some interesting common characteristics. The universal need to set basic goals, policies and strategy was clearly indicated along with the 'typical' set of management functions such as arbitrating on resource allocation, seeking and giving information and motivating others directly and indirectly. A general manager's job is basically seen as very demanding and stressful with the key to the nature of these pressures being the great diversity of complex issues which must be dealt with in a very short timespan. Other jobs of course experience similar pressures but it is the potential involvement in all issues of short, medium and long term duration that particularly characterizes the general management function.

We discussed earlier the precarious distinction between so called goal-orientated managers and those more concerned with process. In the NHS the process-orientated manager has become rather maligned as unconcerned with outcome. It is instructive therefore to consider that Kotter's group of successful managers are preoccupied in their daily behaviour with so called process activities (mainly talking with others, usually briefly and in an unplanned way seeking to influence others and their activities).

They are of course attempting to utilize their power to structure the agenda of the organization as well as maintain and extend their network of influence. These activities are very much concerned with achieving outcomes but are vital 'processes' requiring high levels of interpersonal skills which should not be underestimated. In addition to Kotter's work, some other academic enquiries into the nature of general managerial activity have become minor 'classics' in management studies. We will conclude this section with a brief review of these studies. A major conceptual tangle for all researchers in the area of organizational performance is that of defining an appropriate measure of organizational performance. Each organization will evolve particular performance criteria and it is a contentious issue as to just how clearly managerial behaviour can be judged to be causal in terms of these criteria. A typical solution to the complexity of these inter-relationships is to obtain some form of internal consensus or judgement about 'good' managers in the organization. The work of Mintzberg (1975) and Stewart (1982) are two major and influential contributors to our understanding of managerial work.

Stewart has devised a conceptual framework for examining managerial work comprising.

Demands   – the content of a job that simply must be done in order for the functioning of the organization to continue

Constraints   – the pressures, both internal or external, which place limitations upon what the specific job-holder is able to do (technological, resource or attitudinal limitations)

Choices   – the area where the manager may have some latitude to decide about what or how things are done, including changing an organization's orientation.

The framework provides a particularly useful approach to examining differences in the degree of choice available to managers which typically increases with higher levels of management.

Subsequent work by Stewart (1985) focused upon what managers did with their time. This study enabled her to differentiate the following types of manager.

Emissary   – primary activity is to represent the organization to the outside world and therefore spend little time in the office

Writer   – such individuals are often in specialist functions and deal with information processing and paperwork

Discusser   – a person with a very wide range of responsibilities who spends most of his/her time in discussion (usually on a one-to-one basis) with other managers

Trouble-shooter   – here the job is unpredictable and reactive, typically dealing with crises and interacting with subordinates

Committee Member   – a formal manager, typically in a large organization and with external contacts.

Our ability to recognize individuals of this type is comforting and allows us to conclude that there are several types of manager rather than a single pattern. However, this is of very limited use in identifying the necessary skills and behaviours required to perform these various roles.

Mintzberg on the other hand suggests that managers can be described in terms of various roles or sets of behaviours which all managers perform. The first set is called Interpersonal Roles and incorporates three sub-sets with the manager acting

1. As a figurehead, by presenting the organization to other groups
2. As a leader in which the manager takes direct charge of a group or activity within the organization and finally
3. As a means of liaison both for internal groups and external contacts.

The second set of roles are referred to as Informational and again have three sub-roles of

1. Monitor – keeping abreast of developments externally in the environment
2. Disseminator – the manager ensures that staff within the organization receive all necessary information – and finally
3. Spokesperson – where the manager is required to present information on behalf of the organization to others.

The final group of Decision Roles have four sub-categories. The first, entrepreneurial, is a key role for general managers in helping the organization adapt to new situations or make the most of market opportunities. Inevitably such innovation cannot always be perfect or smooth and consequent repercussion or reaction must be coped with, thus presenting the second sub-role of disturbance handling. The final two roles have been described in other studies in similar terms such as allocating resources and negotiating between departments as well as with unions.

The role structure presented here has received considerable support from subsequent studies. However, both of the models (Mintzberg/Stewart) provide primarily descriptive rather than explanatory constructs. Whilst it is helpful to be able to describe the sets of activities engaged in by managers it is still a stage removed from determining for particular managers why or how they should go about the specific actions and interventions needed by their organization. In other words, a manager may be well acquainted with the roles he/she is playing or the choices available but still not know what actually makes behaviour effective in his/her own context.

Analysis in later chapters helps to move the analysis of managerial behaviour towards this goal. Our emphasis will be upon behaviour rather than descriptive patterns and thereby focuses upon how managers can meet the demand of their positions effectively.

Methods and approaches when examining general management

As with many areas of research the methods used to conduct the investigation can have important implications for the nature of the resultant findings. Managerial case-studies often present very personal, sometimes glamorous, pen-portraits of successful managers and these can make for entertaining reading. Occasionally, some insights may be gained as to how, in retrospect, a particular problem was handled, although the relevance of some information of this type is dubious. Is it helpful in understanding managerial behaviour to know details of a particular manager's childhood, schooling or life history? For example, if we learn that a highly successful manager happened to spend some time in early life on a farm, what is a practising manager to do – book a farm holiday immediately in the hope of improving his/her managerial skills? Similarly the presentation of highly abstracted lists of management functions such as planning, organizing, controlling and so on are of very limited value to a manager in practice. Since all managers do these things it is self-evident that they do them differently and to different effect. We need to know much more about context, time scale and pertinence of each activity to subsequent events.

Whilst we have been critical of the descriptive accounts produced by Stewart and Mintzberg they do at least represent an important development in the study of management, i.e. the move towards empirical study of managers in action. Nonetheless even within this empirical tradition there are major problems of comparability and assumed commonality. The former problem relates yet again to the lack of an agreed set of definitions or language with which to describe managerial activities. As a consequence each study and list of managerial characteristics may have its own internal consistency but other than at a most superficial, subjective level cannot be directly compared to the next. Hence the proliferation of lists of behaviours, partly overlapping and partly obscured by a semantic uncertainty about whether a specific description is quite the same as described elsewhere.

Furthermore, the second assumption about a common set of managerial skills may or may not be valid. Management in all spheres will probably only look the same if very general abstract terms such as monitoring, controlling or planning are used. If being a health service manager is unlike managing an engineering factory then the knowledge and content of these two contexts will, at more detailed levels, rapidly push the descriptions further apart.

Indeed the whole notion that common management skills exist is attacked by Whitley (1988) in a rather complex but important paper. He suggests three critical features of management research/education in support of his contention. First, unlike most professional areas, there is no established body of managerial knowledge which defines both competence and the essential content of any training that could be seen as a prerequisite to effective task performance. This is because the nature of managerial skills is largely determined by employers and by the market context in which they work. Consequently, it is virtually impossible for an employer to insist on a specified range or level of knowledge as a requirement since these are variable and almost certainly changing. Contrast this with the dominance of the medical profession over medical training content and hence approved entry to practice. Whitley's subsequent arguments stem from this primary point. Managerial skills may be characterized as 'variable, contingent and unstable' and therefore knowledge about them tends not to be invariant or context independent. This basic fluidity in what constitutes managerial skills is emphasized further by their interdependence with particular organizational structures and characteristics. Accordingly, managerial skills cannot be studied in isolation from their context. Moreover, any attempt to do so is ultimately doomed to failure if the overall objective is to provide guidance to individual managers about their own managerial performance. We will argue in later chapters that the need is for a cognitive model of managerial behaviour which enables specific management behaviours and influential environmental features to be appropriately linked.

In building such a model we have been influenced by the work of Hales (1986, 1987) who has been critical of many of the previous studies of managerial behaviour. The initial basis of Hales' concern was that the pursuit of descriptive accounts of what managers do has somehow obscured insights into the more pertinent question of 'what is effective management'. If we accept that managers have a signficant contribution to make towards performance outcomes then we must be interested in effectiveness and for Hales this means asking whether managers do what they are supposed to do. Concentration upon the behaviour exhibited fails to answer the second element of this definition of effectiveness. Our concern is with whether what a manager does enables him to achieve what he was supposed to achieve and what he and the organization intended should occur. Hales structures his attempt to review the literature by identifying five major areas of focus within the research evidence. These are

1. Elements of managerial work
2. Distribution of managers' time between the elements

3. The people with whom a manager interacts
4. Informal elements of managerial work and as 'political sensing'
5. Key themes in the documentation of managerial work such as consistency of pattern versus diversity of behaviour.

Some of the evidence resulting from these studies has been presented earlier in this chapter. To add more and more detailed accounts of the different studies would not greatly clarify the nature of management. Although this is obviously an indictment in itself, there are some conclusions to be drawn and some important lessons to be learned.

Firstly, we have already implied there is considerable diversity or inconsistency in the research evidence. Hales suggests this is due to (a) the nature of the management itself and the huge range of jobs that could fall under the rubric of 'manager' and (b) the range of methods used which predispose certain types of results. For example, questionnaires tend to produce formal work elements whilst observation tends to highlight more informal aspects of a manager's work. The plethora and range of descriptive categories used to describe management makes comparison between studies virtually impossible or meaningless. This diversity seems to be accepted in the literature almost with a shrug of resignation and an acceptance of 'that's the way it is'. One might hope for a rather more positive response of trying to improve the conceptual basis of the categories used and also to refine the definition of who are or what are the jobs that shall form the focus of study. To be fair, there has been some methodological development, though, and one can trace trends such as a movement away from a concentration on describing work elements in a rather static form to a more process-orientated approach. Similarly, the definitive set of managerial categories is no longer sought as a more realistic acceptance of the contingent nature of managerial behaviour becomes more widely acknowledged. In recognition of these two major changes there is also less use of pre-defined categories and application of a greater range of methods within a single study.

Hales (1987) has attempted to investigate his ideas about the interlocking of demands, operations and performance in the management task. The focal group was a number of unit managers in the hotel and catering industry. The methodology chosen attempted to incorporate the various features of Hales' arguments about the true nature of management jobs. These techniques therefore examined (a) the role demands placed upon a particular manager by other staff in the organization i.e. the manager's role set; (b) the manager's own conception of the job and (c) an observation of an individual manager for a full working week. Although the findings are described as tentative there is sufficient data from a comparison of similar management posts to suggest that many of Hales' concerns with research into managerial jobs are justified. For example, for two managers who were seen as of equivalent level and who had received similar training the nature of the demands/expectations of their posts revealed considerable differences in absolute number and type of roles as well as emphasis. One manager worked in a national restaurant chain whilst another was a domestic services manager in a hospital. This finding is interpreted as indicating the very strong contextual impact upon managerial work. The observation data focused upon the amount of time each manager devoted within the week to the various job demands, and the differences between the jobs was illustrated by the apparent concentration upon routine administration and maintenance of the restaurant manager as opposed to the domestic services manager's concentrating on staffing policy issues and greater liaison functions.

The notion of effectiveness was addressed by examining the amount of time managers devoted to the various role demands including those classified as particularly important. The idea here was that failure to attend fully to a key task may well indicate some level of ineffective performance. However, as Hales himself admits, there are great dangers in this tactic since time allocated to tasks may not in itself be a fair measure of whether the tasks are being handled well or not. Some important tasks may, by their very nature, not require a great deal of time and this sort of pattern may well bias results if time is used as an indicator.

Despite these reservations, the study is a valuable advance and its conclusions instructive. It suggests that the character of management is influenced by what is managed. If this is true it may have much to contribute to the debate about the appropriateness of managers from other sectors being appointed as general managers in the health service. Secondly, the data indicates that role demands may be more or less homogenous and ambiguous. Therefore, some managers may inherently have a much more difficult task in meeting expectations placed upon them and indeed in being effective. This again may be a very important finding in terms of the wide belief that managing in the NHS with its range of professions is more complex and unlike management elsewhere.

Furthermore, the research methodologies used by Hales would seem to be very much in line with the latest review of the study of management by Rosemary Stewart (1989). Although Stewart refrains from drawing any final conclusions about a 'best' approach she does comment that studying how individual managers think about their work 'is the most open-ended, potentially the most difficult and the most exciting of the possibilities'. This approach would involve trying to understand the constructs particular individuals use to think about their job and subsequently to trace their origins and their impact upon subsequent work activities. It would also attempt to incorporate complex concepts such as how the behaviour adopted is related to outcome at least in as far as the individual manager, as key actor in the process, sees the relationship. Although Stewart suggests that this approach is potentially the most exciting, she also considers that no clear models exist to allow this to happen. In later chapters we attempt to provide methods of approaching how managers think about their work and relating these to outcomes. However, as a minor diversion before developing our approach it is worth considering the question 'Who are the general managers?' The impetus to general management in the NHS has been examined earlier and we have now considered the nature of general management itself. Inevitably the process of bringing together the need for general management and the tasks to be done is personified in the appointment of general managers. The next chapter will consider how this happened and the results of this process in terms of the managers themselves.

CHAPTER 3

Characteristics of general managers

Who are the general managers?

The ready acceptance and speedy implementation of the Griffiths Report by government reflected the fundamental philosophical stance of the present Conservative administration towards the public services, i.e. the push toward greater individual accountability and exposure to the influences of private sector market forces. The latter aspect found its most obvious manifestation in the recommendation that recruitment of general managers to the NHS should include businessmen and managers from other sectors.

The percentage number of managers from various backgrounds is of course constantly changing as individuals come and go. However, a series of analyses through 1986–88 would suggest that this aspect of the proposals has had limited success at least in terms of absolute numbers. Alleway (1987) reports that of all the District General Managers 61% were from administrative backgrounds, 10.5% from the private sector and 5.5% from the armed services. The rest were represented by a small number from a range of NHS professional groups. At unit management level a similar pattern is revealed although there were variations between different regions. Disken, Dixon and Halpern (1987) surveyed almost 700 units and found 62% from an administrative background, 11% hospital doctors, 11% nurses and very few private sector or military background appointees. Allen and Lupton (1988) examining approximately 900 general managers state that 93 were appointed from business, commerce, the armed forces or other parts of the public sector. Clearly the proportion of managers appointed from outside the service is small even against a background of ministerial pressure to look outside. Salary comparisons may well have accounted for part of the difficulty but perhaps more worrying is the reluctance of young, successful private sector managers to see the NHS as an attractive option.

The concerns of this group may have been well justified since examination of the early leavers from general management posts reveals a fairly high proportion were external appointments. Although the numbers in total were small, such departures often attracted great publicity and many possible suggestions were made as to why this might have happened. An overriding comment was that some outsiders were simply unable to adjust to the organizational culture of the NHS. In particular, the political pressures, the strong public interest and the power of the medical profession were frequently cited

Perhaps more influential than these factors alone was the sense that expectations held by outsiders moving into the NHS were just not appropriate. It was felt that some believed the NHS to be totally inefficient – almost a managerless organization waiting to be taken hold of by a firm manager. In reality, a very complex organization was already being managed by individuals who were equally, if not more talented, than many outside but who because of their traditional administrative role were unable to act fully as managers. The key stimulus of the introduction of general management has been to release this pool of talent into a true managerial context. Inevitably some will have been found wanting by the new demands but on the whole the response of the inside appointments has been commendable. The argument about the mismatch of expectations between new managers from outside and the NHS illustrates again the crucial role of values and expectations in effective performance.

Managers for situations

Many writers (e.g. Hales, 1986; Allen and Lupton, 1988) might suggest that such problems were entirely predictable on a theoretical basis. As proponents of contingency theories of management they would argue that managers are more or less effective according to the circumstances and that management skills are not universally transferable. Therefore the dominant caring values of the NHS may have been sufficient to negate skills developed in more authoritarian, efficiency oriented, market-place led organizations. The pervasive values are not necessarily good or bad but they are different, and managerial styles may not transfer readily from one to another. Some external managers have, of course, been successful and this is to their credit in coming to understand quickly the new demands and adapting their approach appropriately. It is also quite possible that they have managed to influence their sector of the organization toward their own preferred style. Movement from both sides is always a possibility. The key aspect to grasp about this situation is that the culture of an organization is not immutable but that success of an individual manager lies in producing a match between the two sets (his/hers and the organization's) of values, attitudes and beliefs which make up the organizational culture. The models discussed in later chapters suggest how a manager can analyze and understand how he/she and the organization relate in terms of cultural compatibility.

Further evidence for believing that there may be significant differences between private and public sector organizations which have a real impact upon managerial practice comes from Solomon (1986). She surveyed nearly 250 senior managers in the different sectors and reported key differences in three particular areas.

1. **Reward systems** Rewards were much more closely associated with performance in the private sector and satisfaction with these policies was also much greater.
2. **Efficiency oriented methods** Techniques associated with more efficiency

such as methods of improving task clarity and task autonomy were more prevalent in the private sector.
3. **Job satisfaction** Levels of satisfaction with the job and with the organization were much higher in the private sector.

It is seductive to believe that importing such factors to an organization like the NHS must be of benefit to both the managers and the organization's own goals. However, this is where the subtlety of culture plays a crucial part. Whilst greater efficiency would not be opposed (except it often means more patients being seen and therefore greater use of resources, and therefore cost) the notion that this is linked to pay rewards for staff is seen as inappropriate and to some individuals almost offensive. This might be a practical version of the culture value clash, where utilizing financial incentives to produce greater throughput may be in conflict with the 'quality' values of the organization and of individuals within it.

Yet another indication of the criticality of obtaining an appropriate match between managerial skills and the organizational context is provided by Gillen and Carroll (1985). They accept the proposition that the impact of managerial skills and behaviours upon effectiveness will vary between situations and are concerned to define just what some of these situational variations might be. Their study focused upon the concept of organic versus mechanistic organizational structures (i.e. the more organic organizations having less defined chains of communication, less definition of job roles and related procedures and greater reliance upon open interaction). In analyzing over one hundred organizations they demonstrated a clear difference in the impact of managerial behaviour upon unit effectiveness. The relationship is much stronger in the organic units than in the more mechanistic ones. This is not to say that managerial performance had no impact elsewhere but that there was more scope in organic units for managerial skills to exert influence, particularly in terms of a greater sense of autonomy and subordinate participation in decision-making. An interesting interpretation of such a finding is that the assignment of managers to particular positions should take account of the repertoire of skills the manager may have in order to capitalize on the opportunities in an organic unit or conversely to bolster a less capable manager by providing the supports inherent in a more mechanistic unit. There may be some important implications here about the problems some managers have experienced in moving from external organizations into the NHS with its multi-constituency groupings of senior professionals.

The discussion in this chapter has attempted to point to the complexity of determining managerial effectiveness by illustrating the interactions with context or situation. It has been assumed throughout though that managers are important to organizational success and that they do have a real impact. Nowhere is this contention supported more strongly than in the bestselling management book *In Search of Excellence* by Peters and Waterman (1984). Fundamental to almost all of the key attributes that they list (see below) is the concept of culture and the role of managers in creating, sustaining and adapting the values and beliefs within an organization that make up this culture.

1. Bias for action, i.e. do it, fix it, try it
2. Closeness to the customer, i.e. listen intently and regularly to the customer
3. Autonomy and entrepreneurship, i.e. innovation and risk taking are an expected way of doing things
4. Productivity through people, i.e. employees are seen as an important source of quality and productivity
5. Hands-on, value driven, i.e. basic philosophy of the organization is well defined and articulated
6. Stick to the knitting, i.e. stay close to what you do well
7. Single form lean staff, i.e. structural arrangements simple, with small head-quarters staff
8. Simultaneous loose–tight properties, i.e. centralized control of values, but operational decentralization.

Implicit in this cultural emphasis is the role of communication in management skills. Clearly the personal attributes and skills a manager brings to the role are likely to be crucial in determining (a) the style in which the managerial task is approached and (b) perhaps the likely eventual success. It is important to ask then what we know about the personal qualities of general managers.

The personal qualities of general managers

For many years, a confusion has existed between the terms leader and manager. In some instances the job specification for the appointment of a general manager has included the term 'must be a leader' as if it was some sub-quality of the concept of manager. This would of course be in direct contrast to those who view leaders in terms of the 'great man (woman)' concept where someone possesses such outstanding qualities that they will emerge as leaders in any context. Leaders must have power and authority and exert influence over others. Zaleznik (1977) suggests that society whilst valuing the role of leaders is also anxious about the potential investment of such power in single individuals. For this reason he believes the collective management ethic has evolved and functions partly as a protection to individuals and organizations. He suggests that in essence management is about problem solving whatever the specifics of the situation or context. From this stance he contends that 'neither genius nor heroism are required to be a manager, but rather persistence, tough-mindedness, hard work, intelligence, analytical ability and, perhaps most important, tolerance and goodwill'. Zaleznik argues that managers and leaders are very different kinds of people, and that these differences may be witnessed in four particular spheres.

1. Attitudes towards their goals – managerial goals are deemed to be essential and created by the organization. Therefore managers can adopt a fairly detached, impersonal attitude toward their goals. In contrast, leaders are active in shaping the goals and influencing others towards them.
2. Conceptions of work – managers are primarily enablers, negotiating and

flexible in their efforts to direct resources towards stated goals. In contrast, the leader though is not willing to operate within the defined realm but rather seeks to change expectations and alter horizons. The propensity to risk is far greater.
3. Relations with others – managers prefer to work with others, often avoiding solitary activities. However, these relationships although numerous are often relatively superficial and confined to the role relationships existing within the organization. Leaders on the other hand seem to produce a more intense and powerful reaction, sometimes of course creating high levels of motivation and at other times a rather disruptive waste.
4. Attitudes towards self – managers tend to see themselves as fitting the world or institution in which they function and playing a role to harmonize and fulfil the expectations of members of the particular community. Leaders however are likely to feel more alienated, as if they do not truly belong to the world or organization of which they are a part. They are thus often propelled towards change.

Kotter (1982) explores this theme further and resolves any conceptual tension by asserting that general managers must act as leaders and in three very particular ways. Firstly, they must have a vision of purpose and goal, secondly, they must be passionately committed to communicating it throughout the organization and thirdly, they must provide the resources for the organization to implement and achieve this goal. It is interesting to note that a current management guru, Charles Handy, writing in 1989 strongly endorses the first of these factors (vision). He writes 'A leader shapes and shares a vision which gives point to the work of others.' In elaborating this he outlines some key principles. The vision must (a) be different; (b) make sense to others; (c) relate to the work other people do and (d) must be understandable. A leader must also be aware that the achievement of the vision depends upon the input of others. For Handy, then, this is the fundamental way in which managers must act as leaders.

The ways in which general managers perform this role may vary a great deal resulting in the complex issues of defining leadership style. Rarely will leadership be expressed through a single and unwavering style. It is far more likely that any individual will call upon many different influencing modes. Some broad categories of leadership style may be identified, such as leading through charisma where some magnetic charm arouses extreme forms of loyalty and enthusiasm. For many, rather more attainable styles might involve utilizing an organization's mission or goal as a rallying call, or negotiating and bargaining with key staff for commitment.

Obviously the choice of style will partly be dependent upon the situation but an equally if not more powerful interacting force will be the individual's personal characteristics. This line of argument has been pursued and examined by Kotter in his intensive study of fifteen general managers. In an earlier chapter we criticized some of the biographic outcomes of this study as not being particularly helpful in understanding how general managers might be developed. Specifically Kotter's discussion of life-history patterns of general managers is difficult to accept. For example one major finding was that almost all the general managers were given relatively early experience of responsibility and fairly high-level posts. Whilst this is true there must also be many who were also given such early responsibilities who did not emerge as successful. Furthermore the self-fulfilling prophecy of early success leading to high self-esteem, high self-confidence and high expectations from others cannot be dismissed. Nonetheless some rather more instructive outcomes are worthy of consideration. Basic personality factors that emerged as themes from Kotter's study may be listed as achievement orientation relating to power, ambition, emotional stability, optimism, intelligence, analytical ability, intuition, a personable style and an ability to relate easily to a broad set of business specialists. These have been collected by Kotter under several major headings. In examining these a little further we have our first set of personal characteristics for the identification and selection of general managers. The categories were as follows.

Knowledge and skills

Managers typically have bright, quick, adaptable minds. This is not to advocate the necessity of intellectual brilliance but certainly above average general intelligence. This must be linked to a very thorough knowledge of the industry in which the manager operates.

Commitment

Ambition and dedication are essential. The job demands though are so great that good physical and mental health is another key quality. This relates to another factor of resilience. Managers have to be able to learn from their mistakes but also to meet up with failure and 'bounce back'.

Integrity

The source of this term stems from the development of trust in an organization, although it is an extremely difficult concept to operationalize. In reality managers may be viewed as possessing integrity through a series of actions over time which engender trust in their staff. There is an obvious tautology here in that actions that lead to trust lead to a manager being described as possessing integrity and therefore capable of inspiring trust. The difficulty inherent in this sort of term is most evident in a selection context where it is virtually impossible for the characteristic to be judged at a single point in time. Similarly, other qualities such as 'presence' and 'judgement' cannot be disputed in terms of appropriateness but are equally abstract and potentially difficult to assess. Once again a manager may only exhibit judgement in dealing with a number of issues over time. Even here the manager's analytic skill may have been sound at a particular point in time but be proved inappropriate by external events.

Concern for others

Managers clearly depend upon co-operation from others, and failure in this area whether due to arrogance or clumsily manipulating others is a frequent cause of problems for general managers.

This listing of qualities from Kotter has been influential in the specification of prerequisites for general management appointments. Despite being
intuitively appealing there are, as we have seen, still many weaknesses
in actually operationalizing such terms. Part of the problem is that the
descriptors used are too general and open to interpretation.

At a much more constrained and specific level Kable (1986) has identified
ways in which managers may differ in their approach to a particular part
of their job, i.e. how do managers make decisions? The technique used
is called *decision perception analysis* and suggests that the way managers
approach decisions can be described as preferences along two dimensions –
quantitative and qualitative. Kable identifies the following categories of
managers.

1. An authoritarian, decisive accountant, serious and formal in relationships
   with other people, analytical but practical, with a dominant personality
   favouring the rule of law (regulations and procedures). This would reflect
   a highly quantitative approach.
2. A sensitive and flexible, friendly personnel manager, supportive of his/her
   people and responsive to people-oriented problems, with an open communicative style. This would be described as highly qualitative.
3. A well adjusted, honest, marketing manager attentive and confident in
   his/her job with balanced but firm opinions and the courage to support
   independent conclusions. This is the combined group being both quantitative and qualitative.

Kable suggests that the frame of reference operating is unique to every
individual manager but considers that matching this individual frame to job
requirements will lead to the most effective decision making outcome. As we
have advocated strongly in these early chapters and as Kable reiterates 'the
real trick is in the matching process'.

It may be possible to approach this matching process from the perspective
of management development. Determining the content of management
development programmes necessarily involves identifying and articulating the
sorts of skills and qualities they should possess. It is then of course up to the
organization to decide just how such skills should be fostered and then to locate
managers in appropriate settings where maximum use of the skills can be
obtained. The writing of Burgoyne and Stuart (1976) is a good example of
the value of this developmental approach. They suggest that a manager at work
is acting upon his/her environment by carrying out 'inner plans' with some
purpose in view. At the same time the manager receives information from the
environment which is about the surrounding circumstances and changes in
it. Effectiveness will therefore be determined by the appropriateness of the
plans and purposes both to each other and to the situation. The model outlined above is a forerunner of the approach described in more detail later in
the text. Burgoyne and Stuart suggest a range of characteristics that are required
to operate successfully within this model of management activity. When the
model was listed by relating the qualities to rated managerial performance the
following pattern emerged.

Successful functioning at senior management level requires

1. Mental agility – grasping a range of problems quickly
2. Productivity – an inclination to respond positively to goals and targets
3. Emotional resilience – maintaining a sensitivity to events and being able to work under pressure
4. Command for basic facts – an awareness of the state of play/people and the organization.

Fast track movement through an organization was additionally reported as requiring

5. Creativity – to come up with new approaches personally and to recognize good ideas from elsewhere and to develop them
6. Analytical, problem-solving skills – ways of deciding effectively between alternatives.

A final factor in this second group was good professional understanding. It is perhaps significant that this was related to fast progress through the organization but not actually required to operate at senior management levels.

In the search for the personal qualities of managers we are in danger of replicating the problems of defining managerial tasks, i.e. a plethora of lists creating a cloud of semantic confusion. Indeed the difficulty is so acute that Hirsh and Bevan (1988) have devoted an entire text to exploring this issue of language use in describing management qualities. Over forty organizations from a range of sectors were surveyed to see what terms were used to describe management qualities. Whilst job-related knowledge did occur, the majority of the lists obtained used a combination of skills terminology (technical skills, interpersonal skills), competencies (running meetings, delegating tasks) and personal attributes (self-confidence, ambition, etc.). The analysis carried out has certain inherent difficulties such as simply counting the number of times a word is given which tends to over-represent common-parlance terms like communication. An alternative approach of looking for key clusters also leads to emphasizing areas where a series of alternative forms exist to express the same concept, and thus such items tend to appear very often. However, given these problems the results are still of interest and the most common items of both methods are presented in table 3.1.

Although the analysis suggests that terms like communication are used fairly consistently, other terms are much more variable. Flexibility, for example, can be a personal attribute or can be applied to thinking style. Predictably, the greatest confusion surrounded the concept of leadership. It can be a collective for all the other attributes or a sub-element of a personal quality, whilst yet others view it as a competence.

A range of methods (including brainstorming, job analysis) and consultants were involved in the original derivation of the lists. Although no single method or approach can be recommended as superior, the general and worrying finding was that very, very few lists had been subject to any studies of predictive validity. In almost all cases the best that could be said is that the descriptions possessed face validity, i.e. they looked as if they were relevant to the type of work and behaviour required by the organization. It is a pity

Table 3.1   *Common managerial descriptors from Hirsh and Bevan (1988)*

Commonest individual words	Commonest cluster of meanings
Oral communication	Managing people
Leadership	Communication
Judgement	Intellect/conceptual
Initiative	Job performance
Organizing	Organizing
Communication	Motivation
Motivation	Specific skills
Analytical skills	Self-confidence
Professional/technical skills	Judgement
Planning	Influence
Innovation	Innovation
Appearance	Stability
Interpersonal skills	Personality
Experience	Career outlook
Numeracy	
Maturity	

that with the resources and opportunities available more evaluation studies have not been undertaken. This might result at least in a significant reduction in the length of the lists. One possible approach which may be of use in disentangling the morass is to try to operationalize the different levels of managerial activity. It is clear for example that certain skills or qualities become more important with increased seniority. Rather than list them at the initial selection stage it may be better to indicate at what point in the manager's progress they can become relevant. This would also make promotion decisions and related development programmes more specific.

Recruiting managers into the NHS is where we began this chapter and clearly one use of the lists of personal qualities presented here is in the selection process. The authors have been heavily involved in this process of recruiting general managers and the final section presents an account of this work and of the key personal variables that emerged as critical to success in the appointment stakes.

Recruitment of general managers into the NHS

In the recruitment of general managers considerable attention has focused upon personal attributes partly because at senior levels technical skills are often assumed. Also, as we have seen, so much of the managerial role involves people and those personal qualities which facilitate these skills are seen as at a premium. The majority of posts in the NHS were filled via rather traditional procedures involving an application form and a formal panel interview. However, more innovative approaches incorporating the use of assessment centre techniques were utilized in some Districts. The authors were involved in many of these and it is this sample that forms the basis of the data reported here.

Assessment centres have increased in popularity very quickly in recent years. A true assessment centre has certain key features such as the use of exercises designed to assess performance on tasks known to be part of the job and derived from a job analysis of the job in question. In addition, trained observers are used to assess the qualities of candidates on a range of activities such as group discussions as well as various forms of interview. Another common element in assessment centres is the use of psychometric lists to assess a range of personal characteristics. All the various exercises are used to obtain a 'rounded' view of the candidate in terms of how far he/she possesses the qualities deemed important to the post. On the whole assessment centres fare very favourably when compared to other selection techniques in terms of predicting job performance. This again has enhanced their popularity despite a relatively higher running cost.

Within the NHS, the assessment centre approach was used which incorporated to varying degrees the features described above. The data described here are derived from the use of psychometric tests within these events.

During the two year period 1984–86 a random sample of 177 short-listed applicants for UGM posts completed the Occupational Personality Questionnaire (OPQ) – Concept Model 3, as part of a wider selection event. The OPQ is a self-report questionnaire which is particularly suitable for occupational uses and has been designed for selection and counselling uses at a managerial and professional level. The item content aims to be direct and work related and measures some thirty personal characteristics. The age range of sample group was between 35 and 50 with 152 male and 25 female. The dominant occupational groupings within the applicant groups were administrators (54%), nurses (16%) and private sector (12%). Of the total group 42 were successful and 135 were unsuccessful candidates. The analysis sought to determine whether there were personal qualities which distinguished between these two groups.

There were relatively few single dimensions that could be said clearly to distinguish the two groups. This is not altogether surprising since, as we have seen, management is in itself an extremely difficult concept to tie down. As a consequence it would perhaps be naïve to expect managers to be recruited on one or a few key attributes. Clearly a whole range of attributes in different combinations may be needed to perform the range of managerial tasks. Indeed when this approach was adopted of looking for clusters of factors some clear differences between the successful and unsuccessful groups became apparent. Successful candidates appeared to be more

1. Directive in their influencing style which in itself was associated with a capacity for decisiveness
2. Independent, holding strong views whilst being good at challenging assumptions and probing issues
3. Successful candidates seemed able to cope better with pressures and also to be more controlled emotionally
4. Comfortable with groups and willing to share views with others, which perhaps surprisingly was itself coupled with a strongly practical, pragmatic outlook
5. The probing, challenging style already mentioned in 2. was also found again to be linked to a relatively tough and resilient personal approach.

It is not difficult from the characteristics listed above to see why such individuals may have emerged as successful candidates. The need now of course is to trace through the job performance of such appointments and relate over time the personal attributes with achievement in post. If such clear evidence can be obtained then the option for improved selection becomes apparent.

It is clear from this chapter that there is no shortage of data on the personal attributes of general managers, but on the other hand there is considerable confusion as to what these key aspects are. Some of this results from confusion of language but much is due to the diversity of management posts and the range of contexts in which they occur.

We move now from considering management and managers to an examination of how they function within an organization and in particular an organization in the process of change.

CHAPTER 4

Understanding organizational change in the NHS

The new general managers in the NHS have a simply stated objective of implementing general management. It has been argued that this is broadly equivalent to promoting change in the organization. Our view is that the manager's mental model of the 'shape' of the new organization and how it gets there is vital to this process. In arriving at an understanding of the factors involved in these models, it is essential to examine what is known about organizational change. Therefore, in this chapter, we turn to the existing research and the many models of the change process which have been proposed.

Any consideration of organizational change can be usefully viewed from two different but complementary perspectives. Firstly, organizational change may be viewed from the 'objective' perspective of explicit theories of organizational change as represented in the ever-expanding literature devoted to the subject. Secondly, organizational change may be examined from the 'subjective' viewpoint of how organizational structure and dynamics are represented in the minds of those individuals involved in the process of change. Both viewpoints are useful and an examination of organizational change should take account of the twin perspective of both explicit organizational theory and implicit, subjective 'theory'. In using the metaphor of theory we are not implying that the implicit subjective theories which managers hold have necessarily been well formulated, structured and articulated. Often a manager's subjective theories of an organization may be fairly loosely defined and structured and compared to the so-called 'expert' body of knowledge may be more or less idiosyncratic. Despite these deviations from textbook theory and variations between managers themselves, the managers' subjective constructs of the organization and the way in which these are related to expectations of change are complex networks of meaning through which organizational events and states are viewed and interpreted.

The extent to which the implicit theorizing of managers may be seen as 'correct' or 'incorrect' is a complex issue but at some level of analysis it seems reasonable to assume that there should be some degree of correspondence between a manager's implicit theory and some aspects of explicit theories of organizational change. If this were not the case the validity of either or both may be called into question. There has been little work on directly investigating the correspondence between implicit and explicit theories of change, although there has been a broad-based attack on many of the issues surrounding the problem of implementing organizational change. This effort has produced a rich crop of ideas but has not resulted in any one complete or coherent theory.

Often it seems that the sprawling literature on change staggers unsteadily under its own weight of contradictory and confusing theories, models and metaphors. This of course means that the correctness or otherwise of managers' implicit theories cannot be simply validated by recourse to a comparison with the explicit theories of organizational change. The situation is complicated further when we are forced to consider the different roles and functions of theory itself in a little greater depth.

Egan [1985] has drawn a useful distinction between explanatory systems 'models' and working 'models' in discussing the promotion and management of organizational change. This distinction is similar to the distinction between explicit and implicit theories of change introduced above. Explanatory models are essentially explicit theories of change. In contrast, Egan (1985) suggests that the 'working models' enable the user effectively to achieve concrete and specific goals within the practical constraints and opportunities of the organization. These working models are characterized by two criteria. Firstly, they must be complex enough to account for the reality they attempt to portray and secondly, they must be simple enough to use.

These 'working models' are practical models which Egan suggests provide a vehicle for translating theory and research into a 'visualization' of how things work. In other words they are assumed to constitute a framework for action and intervention. In an earlier discussion, Legge (1984) has suggested that many of the explicit theories and models of organizational change can be seen as falling either into the descriptive or prescriptive 'camps'. The descriptive approach to organizational change attempts to describe how and why organizational change actually takes place by modelling and diagnosing the dynamics of this process. In contrast the prescriptive approaches to change attempt to provide a specification of how best to achieve different future organizational states or outcomes. They are literally prescriptions to managers of what to do to make change happen, although some have a more 'cookbook' flavour than others.

The correspondence, between formally stated explicit theoretical and practical approaches to change, with subjective informal theories and models of change, which a manager actually uses in attempting to change an organization is of central importance in any attempt to evaluate the change strategies which a manager adopts. Unfortunately, often there appears to be little compatibility.

Current perspectives on organizational change

The main purpose of this review section is to introduce and discuss several prevailing orientations to organizational change and to relate these to the management of innovation in the health service. The early dominance of comparative structural approaches and their roots in 'classical' organizational theory are touched upon, and this traditional approach is contrasted with the emerging longitudinal process perspectives of organizational change.

The distinction between descriptive and prescriptive approaches is used to sharpen the comparison between how change actually takes place and how many feel change ought to take place. The lack of compatibility of the two perspectives has often resulted in a great deal of confusion. This has been exacerbated further by the welter of variables which have been invoked as a means of understanding the life of an organization as it develops and adapts. This plethora of concepts, models and theories serves to highlight the importance of providing general managers with relevant theoretical frames of reference from which they can develop practical 'working' models of the complex systems which they are attempting to change. Unfortunately the enormous variations and permutations of size, structure, culture and function make specific generalizations from the literature difficult to make with any degree of confidence. However, despite these difficulties, there are underlying themes in the literature of change and these are briefly discussed and integrated to provide a framework through which to consider the many and varied issues which a general manager should be aware of in making the transition from theory to practice.

Various common dimensions can be overlaid upon the different perspectives of change apparent in the literature. As we have seen some approaches are primarily descriptive whereas others are mainly prescriptive; some approaches stress slow transformation whereas some stress fast transformation; some approaches focus on organizational structure whereas others examine process; some approaches are essentially behavioural whereas others adopt a social or cultural stance.

As an heuristic device, these dimensions can be usefully employed to broadly categorize current models of change, although often we are still in a 'grey area' where models and categories remain ambiguous. The organizational development (OD) approach, for example, is essentially a prescriptive approach which is explicit and emphasizes fast organization transformation through the facilitation of processes which are seen to occur as a result of change agents' behaviour. In contrast, Cohen *et al.*'s well-known 'garbage-can' model of decision-making (1976) is a descriptive approach where the implicit intentions of people and the social and cultural backdrop of the area are seen as the critical explanatory features. In contrast to the OD approach, this model does not directly deal with speed of transformation or the structure/process dimension.

Of course, absolute distinctions between the 'poles' of these dimensions are rarely found since they reflect continuums of those theoretical or practical ideas which particular commentators on change have selected for consideration. As discussed above 'pure' descriptive or 'pure' prescriptive models rarely, if ever, actually exist since most approaches contain various mixtures of both elements. Similarly, organizational structure and organizational process, like the remaining dimensions cannot always be simply contrasted. However, despite these caveats different approaches have a tendency to emphasize a selection of contrasting aspects of the issues they choose to focus upon, and these differences in emphasis provide the means whereby they can be roughly classified.

Clearly, those who are concerned with planning, designing and implementing change will be drawn to the prescriptive approaches of whatever complexion although one must be aware of the frequent 'cookbook' flavour which is not always theoretically sound. Conversely, the descriptive approaches often appear to be theoretically orientated, over-academic and impractical. As in so many areas there is a gulf between theory and practice which requires bridging. A good theoretical analysis of organizational change does not necessarily lead to good design of change programmes, although combined with sufficient management insight and flexibility to tailor its ideas to the practical context it can prove of greater benefit than a rigidly adhered-to prescriptive solution. Ideally, of course, 'both descriptive and prescriptive approaches should be compatible and reflect a common understanding of the process and management of change. This common corpus of knowledge is not yet available.

The following sections of this chapter review recent approaches to change although intentionally this has not been tackled in an exhaustive manner. Rather, a summary of the major themes and issues has been selected on the basis of relevance to general managers in the NHS and to their central practical concern of what must be done to facilitate necessary changes in the service.

The review is partitioned into three sections, descriptive perspectives on change, prescriptive perspectives on change and cultural perspectives on change.

1. In the first section, four areas are considered: organizational structure, planning and decision-making, the systems dynamics of change and organizational inertia.
2. Section two reviews prescriptive change perspectives, specifically the organizational process approaches of organizational development and 'expanded' change theories.
3. The third section examines three related cultural areas: culture and cognition, cultural change within the NHS and strategies and potential for change.

General managers have become increasingly aware of the potentially con-straining effects of organizational inertia on the implementation of planned change programmes and those factors which are considered to sustain organizational continuity are subsequently discussed. The force of these factors can be traced back to the organization's past structure, culture and history. Examining the role of these antecedent conditions has be-come the main concern of the 'expanded focus' of many contemporary change theorists. This new perspective and its limitations are discussed in relation to the supposedly 'restricted' focus of many OD interventionist strategies.

However, before we examine prescriptive recommendations about what should be done to manage programmes of change, it is necessary briefly to review descriptive or explanatory models of organizational change. As Legge (1984) has pointed out, the value of examining what actually takes place when change is planned and implemented stems from comparing what 'is' with what 'ought to be'. Prescriptive strategies of change are not always derived from descriptive ideas about how the organization actually behaves. This may lead to over-optimistic misconceptions about the anticipated success of change programmes. As we shall see, the idealistic aspirations and subsequent failures of many early OD interventions can be partially explained in this way.

Descriptive perspectives on change

Descriptive approaches in the literature relating to how change is planned, how change occurs, and how change is constrained is briefly and selectively summarized in this section.

Organizational structure

One fundamental and traditional distinction in organizational studies is that made between structure and process. Since the mid-1960s the dominant theoreticians have preferred to focus their attention on factors relating to structure rather than to process variables. From the structural perspective, the NHS, like all formal organizations, 'is a rationally structured system of interrelated activities' (Clifton-Williams, 1978). In this definition, organizational structure refers to those variables which give 'shape' to an organization and includes such things as allocation of work, levels in the organizational hierarchy and lines of communication and control. In an effective organization these structural factors reflect and reinforce the organization's aims and objectives. One of the main objectives of structural studies has been to investigate the degree to which organizations have possessed 'bureaucratic' features and to link the level of observed bureaucracy with other organizational features.

Historically, the structuralist approach stemmed from the pioneering work of Max Weber (1864–1920), who classified organizations into three types: the charismatic organization (dominated by the leader's personality), the traditional organization (dominated by custom and practice), and the rational–legal organization (dominated by clearly defined goal-oriented values). This third type, often called the 'bureaucracy', was considered by Weber to be a particularly desirable way of organizing administrative systems (the term had not, at that time, acquired its pejorative overtones). The notion of investigating bureaucracy was taken up by many structuralist researchers, and their work has been typified by a dominant structuralist research paradigm. This has tended to proceed by recording a cross-sectional measurement of aspects of organizational structure and relating these features to other factors of interest. For example, Pugh and Hickson (1976) found that as an organization becomes older and larger it tends to become more bureaucratic. In another structural comparison, Nystrom (1979) contrasted rigid bureaucratic organizational structures with flexible matrix organizational structures, and suggested that the former structural type is typical of 'positional' organizations (i.e. those organizations which are characterized by stability and continuity with the past) and the latter structural type is typical of 'innovative' organizations (i.e. those organizations which are characterized by a dynamic discontinuity with the past). Nystrom considers that there is little room for creativity and innovation in a bureaucracy because of the emphasis on rules and procedures.

This emphasis on regulation means that organizational members are more concerned with the means of working rather than the ends or outcomes of their efforts. It may be that the emphasis on procedural rules of this type constraint and inhibit attempts by individual members of the bureaucratic organization to try out and experiment with any of their own ideas. If the organizational structure is highly formalized in this way, then this lack of flexibility lessens the probability of job-incumbents interacting spontaneously with those organizational tasks and activities which would benefit by being accomplished more efficiently and effectively (Bell, 1967). It is interesting to note that this description is very similar to comments found in the Griffiths Report.

In an oft-quoted study, Burns and Stalker (1961) placed firms they had studied along a continuum of very mechanistic to very organic and concluded that organic firms were more suited to change. By 'mechanistic' they meant organizations which were characterized by a number of attributes including the following:

1. Specialized differentiation of functional tasks
2. Precise definitions attached to each functional role
3. Clear delegation of responsibility
4. Centralization of knowledge and decision-making
5. Hierarchic structure of control, authority and communication.

'Mechanistic organizations' clearly have many features in common with bureaucratic organizations. At the other end of the continuum are 'organic' organizations which are characterized by factors such as

1. Tasks seen as stemming from the total situation and defined through interaction with others
2. No limited fields of responsibility
3. Spread of commitment throughout the organization
4. Communication consists of information and advice rather than instructions or decisions.

As with other structuralist approaches, this classification focuses on the types of restrictions placed on people's relationships as a function of organizational structure. Closed, highly formalized structures appear to be less flexible and less appropriate when conditions are changing than informal organic structures. Hage and Aiken (1970) have proposed a similar dichotomy whereby static and dynamic organizations are compared and contrasted. A static organization is identified by high complexity of structure, high centralization and high stratification whereas for a dynamic organization the converse applies. There have been numerous attempts to assess types of organization and one useful summary has been provided by Plant (1987) which uses two dimensions, integrated–fragmented and autocratic–permissive, to distinguish four organizational types as shown in Figure 4.1.

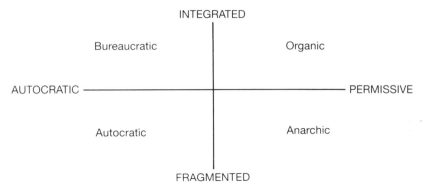

Fig. 4.1 Organizational characteristics (after Plant 1987)

The Bureaucratic organization has the following characteristics: –
Role oriented
Role and status predominate
Communication up and down
Decision made by leader
Answers sought/few ideas offered
Dependence on leader
Moderate dependence on group
Low interaction
High leader satisfaction

The Organic organization has the following characteristics: –
Task oriented
Overall task predominates
Group consensus about decisions
Some shared influence
Solutions sought jointly
High participation/high interaction
More ideas generated
High dependence on group
Share satisfaction – lower for leader.

The 'Autocratic' organization has the following characteristics: –
Power oriented
Power/politics predominate
Answers demanded/rejected
Anti-participation/divide and rule
Withholding of ideas
High integration against leader
Rejection of decision by group
No dependence on group
Low satisfaction to members and leader.

The 'Anarchic' organization has the following characteristics: –
Person oriented
Individual personalities predominate
No decision by group/sharing low

Individual influence
Low interaction/no participation
Possessiveness about own ideas
Individual solutions
Low dependence on group
Individual satisfaction variable.

Despite widespread acceptance of the broad thrust of these distinctions, the structuralists' attempt to derive a coherent theory linking the organizational structure to environmental pressures and internal functioning has not yet resulted in a strong theoretical body of knowledge. This in part results from a pressure to categorize or 'pigeon-hole' very different types of organization even though some of the defining characteristics often do not fit the complexity of real organizations.

This is particularly evident within the NHS when we examine the sharp discontinuity inherent in the advent of the new wave of managerialism. The anticipated consequences of general management's change agendas are partly 'mechanistic' and partly 'organic'. 'Mechanistic' outcomes are evident notably in the areas of increasing the emphasis upon fast decision-making powers vested in the general manager and the strengthening of the hierarchic structure of control, authority and communication. On the other hand there are a number of anticipated 'organic' consequences of general management including expanding fields of responsibility and engendering increased commitment throughout the service.

The extent to which these apparently contradictory outcomes can be simultaneously achieved is debatable. What is clear is that in the attempt to attain them general managers will need to balance the cultural benefits of flexibility and commitment against the structural benefits of authority and control. However, strong theoretical statements of clearly demarcated contrasting organizational 'types' do not seem appropriate to the realities of the emerging structure and culture of the NHS.

Simplistic one or two-dimensional structural distinctions are not adequate in describing the complex and varied NHS environment. In a more complex formulation than the dichotomous approaches of previous researchers, Handy (1976) outlined four kinds of organizational structure and linked these to a particular culture (seen as the climate or 'feel' of the workplace). The four structural categories were classified as pyramid, net, web and cluster and they were respectively associated with role, task, power for success and person-centred cultures. Handy's discussion emphasizes that structures, cultures, and organizational characteristics are mutually interdependent.

Similarly, other studies have suggested that different cultures have different implications for individual and organizational creativity. Nystrom (1979) for example, has argued that creativity is a central concept at both the individual and organizational level and a creative organizational culture is a primary cause of successful innovation.

The fundamental importance of organizational innovation has been widely discussed and variously described, but it is often viewed as a radical change, discontinuous with the past which involves a form of creative problem-solving which is directed toward putting new ideas into practice (e.g. Rickards, 1983). Devising and implementing practical applications of new ideas is seen as the core creative skill in innovation encompassing both the technological and social aspects of an organization. Indeed, the establishment of the NHS itself was primarily a social innovation. The challenge to general management is achieving the balance between organizational stability and innovatory potential, and this is not a simple matter since there is a wide and diverse range of structural and cultural factors which can, depending on local circumstances, either act as inhibitors or facilitators of change.

Effective innovation implies that a general manager is able to maximize change facilitators and to minimize change inhibitors. This in turn, implies that he or she understands what these factors are together with how they can be expected to affect the organization if left unchecked and how malleable they are to imposed change. However, simple causative models are not adequate in describing the process of organizational transformation, and many theorists have adopted a 'contingency' approach in which a large variety of internal and external factors are considered necessary in realistically understanding innovation. A wider conceptualization of change process variables as well as structural variables appears to be crucial, and some of these are considered next.

Planning and decision-making

In a series of case studies, Chandler (1962) studied the strategic change in American firms during the first part of this century. These studies revealed that environmental changes were extremely influential and these external pressures are initially reflected in the organizations' adoption of new products, markets and technology. Subsequently, Chandler found that these initial changes were followed by the organizations' adoption of new internal cultures, structures and systems. Each of the internal changes were made either in response to the demands of the environment or by managerial intervention and these were not isolated but tended to affect the entire system, often in unplanned and unpredictable ways.

Since the early part of the century, the pace of social change has accelerated sharply and this has profoundly affected both private and public sector organizations. For the NHS, external environmental change has been in the form of changing population patterns, public pressure for health care and externally imposed constraints on expenditure. This has prompted the planning and development of new policies and procedures although these very policies have often been criticized.

Planning is frequently described as a rational deliberate sequence of decisions to choose appropriate goals and objectives linked to the actions necessary to achieve them. Much NHS planning has taken place within the framework of this rational model. However, this rational approach is often unrealistic in its expectations since it assumes that decision-making is routine and well prescribed. The uncertainties and vicissitudes of the real world often mean that planning for change is generally an uncertain, ill-prescribed activity. Consequently the desire for rationality in NHS planning can only result, at best, in an exemplar of good planning practice but is more likely to be simply inappropriate.

However, it has been strongly argued that the rationalistic stance is not even appropriate as an exemplar for complex planning and policy-making. Two early expressions of this view came from Lindblom (1959) and Braybrooke and Lindblom (1963) who have argued that complex decisions are not and should not be made by rationally and systematically evaluating alternative programmes but rather by the process of making marginal improvements on the existing state of affairs. In other words, change managers do and should 'muddle through' by making 'disjointed' and 'incremental' decisions. A variation on this theme was proposed by Etzioni (1973) who advocated the 'mixed-scanning' model of planning change in which it is suggested that effective planning proceeds by gaining a broad overview of the main alternatives before scanning the problem at a detailed level. This alternation between the general and the specific results in a series of planning 'stages' and Etzioni's proposed model represents a compromise between clear-cut rationalism and disjointed incrementalism.

In another early attack on the failures of rational planning, Simon (1957) has pointed out that planners do not attempt to maximize rationally the utility of their choices but are content to make choices that are merely 'good enough' to satisfy the demands of the various interest groups who have a stake in the proposed programme (often referred to as 'satisficing' in the literature). Consequently, rationality is 'bounded' and this affects planners' strategies for tackling change. See Cyert and March (1963) for a discussion of some of these strategies.

In yet another criticial reaction to the rationality of many theories of planned change, Cohen *et al.* (1976) have argued that in many choice situations both the planners' goals and how best to achieve these goals are contentious, ill-defined issues. In these uncertain circumstances they suggest that their 'garbage-can' model of decision-making applies. In this model, rather than being regarded as an opportunity for rational problem solving the 'choice situation' may be more realistically seen as

> a meeting place for issues and feelings looking for decision situations in which they may be aired, solutions looking for issues to which there may be an answer, and participants looking for problems or pleasure.
>
> Cohen et al. (1976)

In this analogy decisions occur as outcomes of the interactions of four ongoing contextual 'streams' of problems, solutions, participants and choice opportunities. The model reveals two interesting insights into the process of planning organizational change. Firstly, change is not necessarily problem driven; the solution often precedes the problem to which it may later become conveniently attached. Secondly, the eventual emergence of a programme of change may bear little relation to the explicit intentions of those involved in its planning, but may be presented as 'planned' after the event.

From these various theoretical stances it appears that the rational model of change is unlikely to be able to represent the reality of planning organizational change and becomes less appropriate as change objectives and strategies become more complex and less well understood. Under these circumstances, 'bounded rationality', 'disjointed incrementalism' and the 'garbage-can' analogy may be more appropriate models of how the planning of change actually takes place. The mechanistic rational comprehensive models which typify NHS planning are limiting in their prescriptions and do not appear to be particularly appropriate to the new demands for an innovative organization.

In a recent review of regional strategic planning in the NHS Ferlie and McKee (1988) suggest that scenario analysis could be one useful methodology for tackling uncertainty. As a means of engendering divergent thinking about alternative future scenarios in the NHS, this approach may have some practical value particularly in shaping managers' frames of reference about change and sharpening their understanding of organizational dynamics.

Dutton *et al.* (1983) have suggested that the concepts, beliefs, assumptions and cause-and-effect understandings determine how strategic issues will be framed. From a more academic but related angle, Schwenk (1988) has reviewed four major streams of research on the cognitive perspective in strategic decision-making and highlighted how this research is providing useful insights into the way decision-makers attempt to solve complex strategic problems. The importance of how cognitive frames influence strategic decision-making is becoming increasingly recognized and researched. It has often been observed that the predispositions, preferences and thought processes of top management are crucial in determining the success or failure of business ventures. Many popular accounts of the spectacular growth or spectacular collapse of businesses have focused upon the ways in which the personality and perceptions of the man or woman 'at the helm' has shaped the organizational response. This emphasis upon key individuals in an organization has been receiving increasing support from recent research into the impact of individual organizational perceptions upon strategy formulation. Dutton *et al.* (1983) suggest that strategic issues will be framed on the basis of managers' concepts, beliefs, assumptions, and their understanding of the cause and effect relationships which enable them to 'make sense' of the organization. However, in their attempts to understand organizational problems, managers must typically simplify organizational complexity and in doing so introduce distortions and bias into their strategic assumptions. Schwenk (1988) has described how these strategic assumptions form the basis of the manager's mental model (in the form of cognitive maps or schemata) through which they represent and think about complex strategic problems. The cognitions and internal mental models of key decision-makers are crucial in understanding planning for change and these issues are tackled in greater depth in subsequent chapters.

The systems dynamics of change

The 'systems' perspective is the contemporary credo upon which many articles of management faith are based and itself rests on a number of assumptions. Briefly, the organization is viewed as a system (comprised of a number of constituent sub-systems) which is distinct from, but interacts with, its environment through a series of conversion processes. Because the systems perspective emphasizes input, output and feedback the organization is considered to be very dependent on its environment and change is conceived as a process of adaptation to the environment whereby the sub-systems adjust to maintain the organization's overall dynamic equilibrium. Some of the organizational sub-systems which are frequently discussed are the task, technology, structure and personnel components (Leavitt, 1964). In one popular systems method, the socio-technical approach, two primary sub-components (the social and the technical sub-systems) are seen as being crucial to an organization's effectiveness. By analyzing the relationship between these two major sub-systems the approach aims to diagnose weakness and to reveal areas where the organization's effectiveness may be improved. This approach has been applied to recent work on job design (e.g. Clegg, 1982) and has met with some success.

The popularity of the systems approach stems from its ability to describe the complex interaction of the organization with its environment and to map the interdependence between systems components which can be conveniently defined and redefined in many functional ways. This flexibility of description is useful in suggesting the flow of 'effects' in an organization when one part of the overall system is subject to disturbance or change and 'chains' of cause and effect can be ascertained.

The systems viewpoint is not without its critics however. The nub of the criticism, as Legge (1984) points out, is that by treating organizational members as a component in the wider organizational system, the individual is treated as a passive conformist who is moulded by the deterministic organization and its environment. Like many planning models, the systems approach is seen by many as overly mechanistic. The contrasting viewpoint depicts individuals as actively defining, manipulating and constructing the world in which they live and work.

This active-passive dichotomy is probably more apparent than real since in practice it is clearly dependent upon managers' scope for effecting change. Although resource scarcity in the NHS can be seen to narrow down managerial options for change it can also provide the climate and opportunity for introducing organizational innovation.

Organizational inertia and resistance to change

The proponents of organizational inertia theories contend that change is often a slow, largely unintended and only partially predictable transformation from the old to the new order. Models of slow-moving transformational change suggest that an organization's structure has developed slowly and continues to unfold in a largely predetermined manner. For example, Miller and Friesen (1980, 1984) claim that organizations acquire a momentum which tends to be sustained irrespective of immediate attempts to change the organization's direction. This momentum can be based on previously successful strategies and ideologies and sustained by factors such as standard operating procedures (March and Simon, 1958; Cyert and March, 1963), organizational sagas, myths and ideologies (Hickman and Silva, 1984), single loop learning (Argyris and Schon, 1978) and the interests of political coalitions (Burns and Stalker, 1961; Pettigrew, 1985).

Proponents of this model suggest that successful innovation and change can only occur when the full force of these factors is recognized and the organization is slowly steered in a direction whereby these recurrent forces for continuation have been engineered to flow in the desired direction. This lumbering 'steamroller' view sees the organization as a massive flywheel which cannot be easily stopped or redirected. This emphasis on momentum implies that managers may have less scope for discontinuous changes than they might imagine. Organizational momentum can be based on previously successful strategies and ideologies whose impact and direction can prove extremely difficult to change and which, consequently, inhibit attempts to innovate.

A range of actors inhibit organizational change and attempts to implement new organizational configurations are often met with resistance. This resistance to innovation can significantly reduce organizational effectiveness and if not overcome may ultimately result in obsolescent work methods and skills. However, resistance to change can also exert a positive influence in two ways. Firstly, it may force the advocates of change to build a defensible case and this may avoid ill-advised or over-hasty interventions. Secondly, by limiting the degree of change, resistance can provide a critical stabilizing influence on over-zealous attempts to introduce radical departures from the old order.

Clifton Williams (1978) has discussed reasons why an individual member of an organization may choose to resist change, and highlights such factors as anticipated knowledge or skill obsolescence, fear of job loss, comfort with the *status quo*, peer pressure, lack of information, and limited perspective as some possible causes of this resistance.

Of course, resistance to change can also occur as a group phenomena when internal power coalitions and the micro-politics of organizational conflict are considered. In the widely acclaimed *In Search of Excellence*, Peters and Waterman (1985) examined the influence of political coalitions in organizations and found that their influence may result in a large element of chance about the outcomes of formal organizational decision-making. These unintended outcomes are often the intended consequences of a plurality of intended actions and stem from the very powerful impact of the vested interests of political coalitions. The strength of these political interest groups is often such that any rationalist prescription for planned organizational change will be rapidly subverted. Consequently, many would contend that the analysis of the political systems within an organization is crucial when attempting to implement change – a point also strongly endorsed by Pettigrew (1985) in his study of the political battles in ICI.

In addition to the constraining effects of organizational momentum and micro-politics on proposed organizational change, Stinchcombe (1965) has proposed that there are other powerful processes which act to maintain organizational stability over long periods of time. Part of this ongoing inertia is supported by a 'hidden' form of control in which many 'non-decisions' are made implicitly. This hidden form of control is a 'taken-for-granted' set of rules which is generally outside the arena for negotiation and has been called 'hegemonic control' (Crozier, 1976; Friedberg, 1979). The medical profession within the health service can be seen as holding hegemonic control over a wide range of decisions, which has a profound influence not only upon clinical matters but upon the wider organizational culture and the management process itself.

The ascendency of the medical profession and the knowledge of scientific medicine they possess is being increasingly challenged, not in terms of its clinical validity but in terms of its dominant role in steering health care planning and implementation. The issues of providing health care within an increasingly complex background of resource provision and usage cannot be confidently left to the medical profession alone, and the aim of management must be to bring 'taken-for-granted' rules and assumptions into the arena for discussion and review.

Often the factors which support organizational inertia and momentum are unanalyzed and underestimated and within the NHS, the 'clinical freedom' of the medical profession has been widely recognized as an important source of organizational inertia, although the full strength and extent of clinician's hegemonic control of the service is not yet fully appreciated. Underestimating the power of the medical profession stems from failing to understand the factors which trigger and define the ongoing trajectory of events which link the NHS's history to its unfolding future. Effectively changing the roles and relationships of medics and managers within the NHS requires the application of organizational theory to the problems of implementing change in practice. This application is discussed in many prescriptive approaches and these are subsequently reviewed.

Prescriptive perspectives on change

Organizational process

In contrast to the cross-sectionalist structuralist approach, briefly overviewed in the first section, those who favour a process perspective tend to utilize a longitudinal or developmental approach in their studies of organizational change. Two distinct orientations can be identified within this process perspective. The first orientation is the organizational development (OD) approach which has, until recently, been the dominant process perspective. The second is the newer and rapidly emerging 'expanded' focus on change which adopts a wider, more encompassing view of organizational process. Despite the enthusiastic claims made by its protagonists in the 1960s and early '70s, the OD approach has increasingly received a great deal of pointed criticism. The OD approach adopts a highly rational and linear view of process, which many consider to be restrictively narrow. OD models suggest that organizational processes tend to unfold in a single pre-set direction with minimal parallel developments. Typically, OD practitioners have paid scant attention either to the influential role of key personnel or to the effects of antecedent conditions on the needs, politics and conflicts of organizational members.

In his important contribution to the literature of change Pettigrew (1985) criticizes the rational–linear theories of change presented in OD models. In this author's view, change is not a matter of a rational process of consultation followed by a clearly prescribed step-by-step intervention strategy. Rather, the significance of innovation becomes evident not by viewing change as an isolated episode divorced from the social and historical context, but by reconceptualizing change as a sequence of episodes embedded in an ongoing struggle for power, status and reward.

By considering social, cultural and historical factors, Pettigrew's (1985) approach offers an expanded focus on the simplistic OD models of change and in his case-studies of change in ICI captures the real flavour of change. This 'expanded focus' on organizational change is extremely valuable in capturing the richness and complexity of real organizational change but is itself not immune to criticism in a number of crucial areas, which are discussed later in this chapter.

These two contrasting prescriptive perspectives on organizational change are reviewed in this section.

Organizational development

Kurt Lewin, who in his early research of group dynamics had stressed its theoretical and conceptual formulations, held a positive view of the possibility of organizational change given the 'correct' intervention strategies. Lewin laid the foundation for the OD movement and his three-phase model of change (unfreezing, moving and refreezing) was the key idea in the original emerging formulation of this approach. However, the term OD now covers a multitude of approaches to planned efforts to change organizations.

Kahn (1974) has observed that there is a plethora of OD definitions and this reflects a diverse range of practitioners' preferred approaches in selecting techniques, targets and processes. In his recent attack on OD, Pettigrew (1985) has claimed that OD has as many definitions as practitioners and cites Beckhard's (1969) definition as capturing the idealized vision of OD in the heyday of the 1960s.

> Organizational development is an effort, (1) planned, (2) organization-wide and (3) managed from the top to (4) increase organizational effectiveness and health through (5) planned interventions in the organization's processes using behavioural science knowledge.

A later, more inclusive definition (French and Bell, 1973) proposed that OD could be seen as

> . . . a long-range effort to improve an organization's problem-solving and renewal processes, particularly through a more effective and collaborative management of organizational culture – with special emphasis on the culture of formal work teams – with the assistance of a change agent, or catalyst, and the use of theory and technology of applied behavioural science, including action research.

French and Bell (1973) have provided an iterative sequential model for OD interventions. This planned sequence is considered to comprise the following stages:

1. Initial exploration of the organizational change focus with clients
2. Design of a data-gathering approach
3. Collection and feedback of data to the client group
4. Discussion of the data
5. Action planning
and,
6. Action taking.

Other theoreticians have proposed similar linear phase-management strategies of intervention (e.g. Blake and Mouton, 1968; Margulies and Adams, 1982). In a useful overview, Brill and Pierskalla (1982) have provided a clear summary of OD techniques.

Goal setting Process that usually follows the definition of the organizational mission. The organization defines specific future targets.
Organizational diagnosis Process in which questionnaires and/or interviews ascertain current internal strengths and weaknesses as perceived by organizational members.

Direct observation Process in which a person or persons, usually a consultant, watches key groups functioning in the organization and arrives at conclusions about the organization.

Policy establishment Alterations in the rules that control the organization and its members.

Committee formation Formation of a group to study and/or recommend changes in specific areas of the organization.

Sociotechnical intervention Process of trying to optimize the social and technical fit in an organization.

Team building Process of building cohesion through looking at and/or improving interdependence among various groups.

Communication training Training programmes that help organizational members to recognize factors that affect communication and to communicate better.

Role negotiation Process of clarifying overlapping responsibilities.

The changes sought through OD intervention are generally 'processual' rather than structural and are frequently directed at general rather than specific issues (e.g. the issue might be the organization's problem-solving ability rather than specifically helping to solve any one particular problem). The problem-focus of OD tends to be at the general level of goals, quality of working life and of organizational effectiveness (Bennis, 1969). In its early days the emphasis of OD was centred on improving social skills and interpersonal communication, and this humanistic orientation has often been criticized. Payne (1981) for example, has argued that it is not enough to train people simply to talk and to listen to each other. However effective the communication process can become, the real need is to ensure that communication centres around how the work of the organization can be done more effectively. The rejection of consensus management within the NHS resulted from a realization that endless meetings to facilitate communication and discussion of issues was itself becoming a significant brake on real organizational responsiveness. The problems of the NHS did not primarily stem from interpersonal dysfunction but from weak core management structures and systems of control.

Recently, the emphasis in the OD literature has shifted away from the human-relations approach to stressing the need to match the intervention strategy with the underlying causes of the organization's difficulties. For example, Tichy and Beckhard (1982) have equated OD with organizational design and suggest that organizations are designed and redesigned (i.e. changed) according to the information needs of tasks and the interdependence of tasks. Consequently, one critical function of management is to design organizational structures appropriate to the problems facing the organization whilst instigating successful mechanisms of organizational control. The NHS's concern to identify new general management structures is typical of such activity.

As OD has expanded its boundaries, the diagnosis of the organization's problems and the subsequent selection of an appropriate change strategy has become an increasingly complex process involving the evaluation of many factors. In one application to hospital management, Fry (1982) suggests the following stages.

External analysis Agree on summary of forces placing demands and constraints on hospital.

Internal analysis For each external force decide (1) How is the hospital responding today? (2) What will happen if the hospital continues its present response? (3) What are the alternative responses?

Issue identification and scenario analysis Identify compatible and mutually exclusive alternatives: determine ideal responses not currently being demanded.

Generation of alternatives and analysis and evolution of mission Generate sets of alternative courses of action; determine core mission based on preferred courses of action.

Creation of plan Implement or move toward goals in core mission.

Like many OD prescriptions, this approach can be criticized not only for its failure to confront explicitly the problems of organizational politics but also for its omission to clarify what the underlying 'values' of this intervention might be.

Edmonstone (1985) has discussed the 'values problem' in OD and points out that Organizational Development can be criticized for being 'polluted' by the values that practitioners hold about what problems are worth studying and what questions are worth asking. This problem is exacerbated by the lack of a coherent OD model or theory, the absence of which allows practitioners free rein to exercise their personal preferences not only in the specification of objectives, but also in the selection of problem areas and the application of techniques.

Friedlander (1976) has highlighted the reasons for this diversity in the OD field by identifying the three basic value stances from which OD has been derived. These three stances – rationalism, pragmatism and existentialism – do not rest easily with one another since their associated models, activities and objectives are often incompatible and cannot be easily integrated without conflict. Edmonstone (1985) discusses two possible solutions to the 'values' problem offered in the literature. The first solution entails clearly and explicitly stating to the client the particular set of values inherent in the OD approach. Since this value base typically takes the form of a humanistic stance where personal growth, autonomy, trust, openness and emotional expression are seen as appropriate change outcomes it would seem reasonable to make the client fully aware of these anticipated outcomes. The second solution involves the practitioner developing a more 'value-free' stance in which a less restricted framework of values is used as a basis to view the problems of organizational change.

Consequently, the practitioner can play a more pragmatic role in increasing effectiveness, performance and productivity rather than constantly striving for unattainable visions of the ideal organization.

Whether these supposed 'solutions' to the problems of OD point the way to a realistic development is dependent on whether this approach can acquire greater coherence and identity either as a theory or a profession. Currently OD appears to be 'all things to all men' and this clearly lessens its status as a distinct and practical approach to the problems of organizational change. Pettigrew (1985), as already seen, has severely criticized OD as a simplistic view of change and some of the main thrusts of his arguments are presented in the next section.

The expanded focus on change

Pettigrew (1985) has bemoaned the dearth of studies which attempt to go beyond the restricted analysis of change as an isolated event and begin to examine the how and why of the dynamics of change. The expanded focus which he offers as a supplement to the rational theories of planned change emphasizes not only processual factors but also the historical, cultural and political features of organizational change. Pettigrew's work is both a theory of change and a case study of the process of change.

Pettigrew argues that organizational change should be viewed not as a well prescribed act of intervention but as 'a natural process combining elements of external pressure and internal management action'.

Four important stages are discernible in this 'natural' process.

1. The development of concern by a subset of people in the organization that, possibly as a result of environment change, the present stage of the organization no longer is compatible with its operating environment.
2. The acknowledgement and understanding of the problem the organization now faces, including an analysis of the causes of the difficulties, and alternative ways of tackling these difficulties.
3. Planning and acting to create specific changes in the light of the above diagnostic and objective-setting work.
4. Stabilizing the changes made by detailed and careful implementation plans which include how the organization's reward, information and power systems reinforce the intended direction of changes.

Pettigrew's model suggests that change often originates with a small subset of people in the organization who have become aware of a mismatch between the demands of a changing environment and the current performance of the organization. If change is to be successfully implemented then this new perception of shortfall needs to gain legitimacy. In Pettigrew's view, it is the concept of legitimacy which provides a crucial link between the political and the cultural facets of organizational change. It becomes essential for those who are pursuing the objectives of change to delegitimize their opponents' ideas and actions in order to mobilize concern, energy and enthusiasm which stimulates appropriate action for change. In this necessary delegitimization of the old stance and legitimization of the new perception, the agents of change are not advised to force through an idea against the desires of other interest groups; rather they need to develop the skill of 'intervening in the political and cultural systems of the organization in order to build up a nucleus of political support' (Pettigrew, 1985).

It is clear, then, that change cannot be adequately understood if it is viewed as only resulting from the dictates of management, since management themselves are a key part of the ongoing intra-organizational struggle for power, status and reward. Change occurs not as the result of isolated managerial goal-setting but as the outcome of power struggles between different interest groups.

In his case study of organizational change at ICI Pettigrew focuses on the attitudes, roles and skills of top managers and the effects of social, political and economic change to examine the processes of decision-making and conflict within the firm. It appeared that different change strategies were appropriate to different eras with their differing socio-historic contexts, and distinct change strategies were attempted in different divisions of ICI. The reader is referred to Pettigrew's book *The Awakening Giant* for a detailed discussion of the case studies within each division.

The general conclusions from Pettigrew's case-study approach is that the contribution of the OD initiative was minimal in contributing to strategic change in ICI. The traditional humanistic OD concerns of co-operation, participation and delegation became increasingly cosmetic and irrelevant as the pressures of wage bargaining, new technology and competition became the key factors at the root of real change.

One major problem with Pettigrew's expanded focus on organizational change is that, although the theorizing which permeates the book makes compelling reading, few links are made between this theorizing and his own empirical evidence. The complexity and inclusiveness of the approach means that making predictions about the anticipated directions of organizational change is difficult if not impossible. Pettigrew's (1985) criticisms of the OD approach as 'being all things to all men' would appear to be equally applicable to his own expanded focus on change. The old adage 'there is nothing so practical as a good theory' is as difficult to apply to the simplistic restricted phase-management approach of OD as to the subtle, complex and possibly over-inclusive approach of Pettigrew's 'expanded focus' on change.

Cultural perspectives on change

Culture and cognition

Over the last decade, the ideas of 'organizational' and 'corporate' culture have become increasingly used as a metaphor to understand the ways in which organizations maintain and adapt themselves to internal and external pressures to change. Unfortunately 'culture' is a very yielding word which can be moulded to suit almost any situation. Operationalizing exactly what it may refer to in the day-to-day world of management is not a straightforward task and many now believe that the construct has become so malleable as to be devoid of any practical meaning. This pessimistic stance is probably too sweeping and an alternative view is emerging which, whilst recognizing the dangers of tagging the culture 'buzz-word' to anything vaguely organizational, maintains that the idea itself still has a great deal of usefulness in helping us understand organizations. This very issue is debated in the editorial of a recent Journal of Management Studies. In the editorial Hofstede (1986) argues that the explosion of interest in the organizational culture concept stems directly from a recognition that focusing on individual organizational sub-systems may be less appropriate in some instances than adopting a holistic outlook whereby measures of total institutional strength can be produced. This interest in the broad holistic descriptors of an organization gives an apparently unifying simplicity to the culture concept which has enabled it to be packaged into a number of management best-sellers.

Reflecting and reinforcing the cultural stance has been a concurrent revival of interest in the subjective and emotional meanings of the organization to its members. A number of writers have contrasted the 'traditional' paradigm that organizations consist of objective variables which can be measured by management scientists with an alternative emerging stance which considers that organizations are composed of subjective constructs which are housed in the minds of its members. People's behaviour in organizations may be better understood in terms of their subjective mental frameworks than measuring apparently objective organizational variables. Schon (1971), for example, states

> Thus, whatever might seem to be a piece of direct empirical evidence about an organization's structure (e.g. a constitution, an organizational chart, a job description or a title on an office door) derives its behavioural effect from employee's common understanding and acceptance of its meaning.

Both the cognitive and cultural perspective on understanding organizations are becoming a useful way of considering organizational change. Both stances are concerned with subjective and emotional meaning but whereas the cognitive approach is primarily psychological, dealing with the individual organizational member, the cultural approach is primarily sociological, dealing with shared understanding and common values. Practically an insight into the cognitive and cultural approaches is at the heart of effective change-management.

Cultural change within the NHS

Part of the problem with operationalizing the term 'organizational culture' is that the term 'culture' itself is necessarily abstract. However, the management of change is not in itself an abstract event although it may entail a great deal of symbolic activity. For change to succeed it must rest on a practical and coherent approach which requires a manager to understand what culture he is embedded in and how to apply this understanding in effectively implementing and managing change. In simple terms, it is what managers actually choose to do which counts, although these overt behavioural aspects of management cannot be divorced from the underlying concepts, schemes and mental models which support them. Plant (1987) has argued that the learning process is the key to managing both self-change and change in organizations. This process view sees this learning experience taking place through a number of stages in which the change agent can act either as an evangelist or an educator. Both approaches may prove necessary in the NHS.

General managers in the NHS tend to have an ambivalent view toward the idea that understanding and controlling organizational culture is central to the success of their activities. This ambivalence stems from how they perceive the extent of their power in changing the course of events. On the one hand, taking aboard the ideas surrounding the organizational culture stance appears to open up whole new vistas of possibilities of change. On the other hand, the cultural perspective is often treated with suspicion since it challenges any manager's self-image as a rational, democratic individual. Gagliardi (1986) discusses some of these issues and has highlighted managers' resistance to use symbolic persuasion and ideological suggestion as legitimate instruments of change management. To illustrate the point this author makes the useful distinction between education and propaganda in the management context.

Education appeals to reason and critical thinking while propaganda works on the emotions and the need for identification and certainty. When a leader proposes and wins acceptance for a certain ideology and then uses its cohesive and motivating powers his personal responsibility in doing so is doubtless a real problem which must be faced. However it is necessary to recognize that, to a greater or lesser extent any leader makes use of symbols and values when he manages a regime, even if he is convinced he is managing democratically or 'by objectives'.

It seems clear that rational argument, logical reasoning and negotiation do not always lead to the adoption of new and necessary strategies to solve pressing organizational problems. Many would argue that one of the core problems within the NHS stems from the deeply-rooted and widely-held traditional values of the clinicians within the service. One real problem confronting management is to encourage clinicians to become more actively involved in the management process. This necessitates managers winning acceptance for a new set of organizational values and priorities, whereby clinicians become managerially responsible and accountable for their actions.

Creating these new values within the organization implies that managers need to instigate the process of cultural change. However, in reality, as Greiner (1982) has pointed out, the processes of engendering cultural change have not as yet been fully explored and remain an area open to much debate.

However, two contemporary prescriptively-orientated approaches to change provide some useful signposts for the health-service manager. These two approaches are those of Van de Ven (1980) and Quinn (1980). Van de Ven contends that the target for change should be development and changes of ideas rather than any attempt directly to change people's roles or the organizational structure. Ideas should be selected because of their relevance to problem-solving and top management should focus the attention of different organizational interest groups on the processes of developing and studying these new ideas. To this end, the management tactic should be to 'assist' their colleagues to perceive the problem within the wider context of surrounding issues in order that interest groups can understand and appreciate the full ramification of the problem. Quite understandably, this process can take some considerable time as many general managers have found in their efforts to 'assist' clinicians to appreciate the wider issues surrounding clinical workload, budgets and expenditure.

By first gaining this problem appreciation in other interest groups, Van de Ven suggests that management has already facilitated an introduction to the next stages of the change process. In this next stage, practical collective action can begin to be instigated. This collective behaviour can be motivated and sustained by ensuring the involvement of interest groups so that ultimately institutionalism of the new management ideas takes place. This achievement of legitimacy enables these ideas to become part of the emerging culture.

The approach advocated by Van de Ven suggests an incremental or step-by-step strategy as does the model of 'logical incrementalism' proposed by Quinn (1980). In Quinn's view (*Strategies for Change*, 1980) top management should create the 'logics' which give coherence to the establishment of the change process. This coherence is achieved by gaining broad commitment to the new ideological stance. This requires that top management hold a clear 'vision' of the direction of change, and it is imperative that this vision is transmitted to and accepted by others. Consequently, management should be constantly attempting to use opportunities to promote the acceptance of this vision, although it must be realistically expected that major organizational sub-systems will be differentially responsive to the call for change. The creation of broad commitment is seen to provide the potential for incremental learning in the various organizational sub-systems. Since it is in these sub-systems that the operational details of change will be worked out it is particularly important that any over-specific management guidelines for transformation are not attempted at the sub-system level since specific policies are considered by Quinn to hamper the grasping of opportunities through which personnel learn the new ideological structure.

Both approaches of Van de Ven and Quinn highlight the importance of persuading others to invest information, support and resources into the new organizational initiatives. Strategic and structural change are intimately intertwined and their transformation has to be preceded by ideological changes. The question of how management can begin to instigate these changes in values and culture is considered in the next section.

Strategies and potential for change

In terms of the general manager's strategy for changing the organization he or she needs to be able to understand, predict and control key aspects of the organizational culture. The potential for effective intervention depends upon an understanding of what power he or she has in changing the organization and how this power may be used.

A manager's scope for influencing and directing his organization clearly depends upon a wide range of factors. These facilitators and inhibitors of power have been increasingly debated over the last decade in the management literature. Behaviours and attitudes relating to feelings of 'enpowerment' or 'powerlessness' appear to be extremely potent in determining the sorts of behaviour which people feel may lead to failure or success. From this perspective, the advent of the Griffiths-management philosophy can be seen as primarily a means of enpowering the new breed of management by eroding the perceived necessity for consensus decision-making. Despite these fundamental changes in managerial responsibility, it is still difficult to estimate a general manager's real scope for effective action without examining the wider psychological and sociological processes through which any organization acquires its values. Schein (1984) defines culture as

> The pattern of basic assumptions which a given group has invented, discovered or developed in learning to cope with its problems of external adaptation and internal integration which have worked well enough to be considered valid and therefore to be taught to new members as the correct way to perceive, think and feel in relation to those problems.

This approach is valuable because it sees the creation of the organizational culture as a dynamic learning process although it does not adequately account for those situations when organizations do not abandon deeply-rooted values in the light of experience. Gagliardi (1986) has argued that if a value is deeply rooted in the culture of an organization then it is precisely for that reason that it is not easily cast aside since it is never brought into the arena for discussion and criticism. The idealization of past success generates stable values and ideologies which cannot easily be unlearned or changed.

Within the NHS the traditional status of medical knowledge and the dominant role the clinical viewpoint plays in the design and running of health-care systems are only recently entering into the arena for debate. Whether in practice this means the end of medical hegemony in the NHS depends to a large extent on the strategic interaction of management and clinicians. The on-going power struggles between management and the medical profession will prove to be the key factor in shaping the emerging culture of the NHS.

This type of intervention is illustrated perfectly as the process of implementing the resource management initiative proceeds. Clearly the involvement of clinicians in the specification of the information needed for medical audit and for detailing the activities of a hospital is vital. Nevertheless, despite the quality spin-off that is apparent from better information many clinicians remain sceptical, if not opposed, to the commitment of their time as well as the potential for financial containment which better knowledge of their working practices could produce. Once again managers may be clear about the end point they desire but have to be careful about how they lead, cajole, persuade, request or seek the support of clinicians in this important activity. It is as if the power battle has been presented with a new arena.

Management efforts to delegitimize the prevailing medical grip on planning, policy and procedures will require them to build significant political support so that their interventions steer the political and cultural systems of their organizations in the directions they perceive as appropriate.

The resilience and continuity of organizational culture does not mean that organizational behaviour is repetitive or unchanging. Rather, the implication is that the innovatory potential that an organization possesses is limited. Clearly the positive cohesive and communicative benefits of a common organizational culture must be offset by the potential extent to which that culture can be changed when necessary. Culture can prove to be either a facilitator or inhibitor of organizational change. Whether it is primarily a cause, a consequence, or correlate of change depends on many factors, not least the tactics and strategies a manager adopts.

CHAPTER 5
Mental maps of change

The common focus of change

Since the adoption of the Griffiths proposals, the impact of the new management ethos has been felt to different degrees at different levels throughout the NHS. Despite wide differences and much debate surrounding the selection of change targets, management methods and tactics, those within the new management structure appear to have one fundamental common objective. This objective lies at the core of all the recent attempts to redirect the course of the service. Their common goal is to change the organization from a service which is administered by consensus to a service which is managed by managerial discretion and choice. This fundamental change is aimed at radically transforming both organizational values and the way work is done within the NHS and has been accompanied by a wide range of management initiatives.

These recent initiatives represent a challenge to medical autonomy in a number of ways. The appointment of general managers into the NHS has meant that consensus team-management and the ubiquitous use of the medical veto has ceased. Managers now have the opportunity to challenge medical opinion. Most, of course, will choose this option only as a last resort but the implicit structure has been created. The proposed new contracts for medical staff take this process a stage further.

General managers are increasingly aware that an increased accountability to managerial priorities requires tackling at both the cultural and operational levels. As an example of this dual-pronged approach, consider the many initiatives by which managers are attempting to engender efficiency consciousness with respect to performance, workload and expenditure. These approaches are not merely management cost-containment exercises but are also vehicles to attempt to expand the role of many NHS personnel from simply being the facilitators or deliverers of health care to becoming more responsible to management and more financially accountable for their actions. For example, attempting to develop the managerial role of clinicians goes hand-in-hand with assisting them to expand their organizational awareness to encompass the complex interactions between causes and consequences which characterize any large organization such as the NHS. Specifically, securing systems by which clinicians hold and control budgets could enable greater managerial control over costs and enable the stronger imposition of managerial priorities. From this perspective, the key task assigned to NHS management is to engender expanded and realistic perceptions of organizational objectives together with individual reappraisal of traditional roles within the framework of the new management arrangements.

In striving for this goal of involving a much wider band of participators in aspects of the management process, general managers are trying to break down the traditional boundaries and demarcations between technical, medical and administrative concerns within the NHS. In practice, this is no easy task, and although general managers may ultimately be able to delegate complete budgetary control and responsibility to others, the stumbling block to change may prove to be the entrenched attitudes of clinicians toward what they see as the appropriate role of medical influence.

In a recent paper discussing medical autonomy in the NHS Harrison *et al.*(1989) have highlighted that despite three years of general management, the level of medical influence remains surprisingly high and the lack of perceived impact of the new managerialism appears to be widespread throughout the service. Through a wide-ranging set of interviews with managers, consultants, authority members and nurses, it became apparent in this study that managers were frequently unable to implement particular changes as a direct result of consultant opposition. These obstructions were of two broad types. The first type were called 'overt' and were due to the direct clinical blocking of change initiatives, often accomplished through the machinery of medical representation on decision-making committees. The second type of obstruction was more subtle but equally, if not more, pervasive in undermining the motivation for change. This second 'covert' influence referred to general managers' reluctance to directly challenge or criticize clinicians probably because they have to work with them on a day-to-day basis and feared that conflict could precipitate wholesale non-cooperation.

Although in some districts, those who were interviewed in the study did cite some examples of shifts in the traditional balance of power, it became apparent that there were fundamentally different values which different interest groups hold about the respective roles of managers and medics. The traditional pre-Griffiths perceptions of the manager as a diplomat and the medic as autonomous professional appears to be a deeply instilled stereotype of the NHS psyche, and changing these ingrained perceptions will be a task that requires sustained effort if there is to be a significant transformation of the prevailing culture.

How the organizational structure and the roles of its actors are perceived and represented in the minds of its members has been called the 'cognitive infrastructure' of the organization. This infrastructure includes an individual's internalized model of both the structural components and the process dynamics of the organization. In the final analysis an organization only exists in the minds of its members, and the benefits of positive particpation and shared objectives by those involved in the change process are related to the extent to which they share the same mental model of the organization at any one point in time. 'Real' change ultimately rests in the minds of the people who work in an organization, and from this perspective any organizational intervention can be seen as a means of directly or indirectly infiuencing the way in which an individual perceives the organization and his or her role within it. If organizational change is to be far-reaching and not merely cosmetic, then the manager's vision of change must be reflected in the values, attitudes and expectations of all individual organizational members. If successful, these individual changes in perception of the roles and rules of the organization will form the basis for a collective identification with new organizational values and facilitate the emergence of a transformed organizational culture.

What appears to be of crucial importance to the general management experiment, is the issue of changing the role perceptions of those different interest groups within the system. The management of change rests upon the ability to foster new ways of looking at what appear to be old and apparently intractable issues. This emphasis on the meaning of the organization to its members does not necessarily imply that the targets for change should always be the direct development and inculcation of new ideas, values and attitudes. Rather, implementing successful change strategies should recognize that the transmission and sharing of common frames of reference is an essential element in leading, managing and shaping organization initiatives. These common frames of reference include a relevant shared data-base between managers and clinicians so that the performance and value of clinical activities can be better assessed.

Change agents and activities

The general manager is the key agent of change in the NHS and the responsibility for effective innovation ultimately rests at this senior level. However, since most planned programmes of change fail unless other members of an organization share a common set of objectives and positively participate in change implementation, then it is clear that almost anyone in the organization can act as an agent of change by facilitating progress in the right direction. General managers are obvious change agents but so are their first-line managers, medical staff, nursing staff and potentially anyone else in their charge.

Of course, for any member of an organization to be effective in the role of change-agent, it is necessary that they have at their disposal the appropriate skills and are able to effectively apply these to those organizational situations with which they interact. These change-agent skills are those skills which enable individuals to assess the ways in which various aspects of the organization impact on performance at the individual and group level and on the basis of this assessment to involve themselves positively and creatively in challenging past organizational assumptions. These systems-involvement skills rest upon understanding the current state of the organization and determining effective strategies of intervention. Three broad sub-systems are involved in understanding organizational dynamics; these can be called the work system, the social system and the cultural system. Aspects of these various organizational sub-systems have been frequently discussed and, as we have seen in the previous chapter, often formalized into descriptive or prescriptive organizational 'models'.

In one early but useful 'model', Leavitt (1964) has suggested that any organization is a multivariate system comprising the independent sub-systems of tasks, structure, technology and people. It follows then that any individual acting in the role of change agent can focus his or her innovatory attempts primarily on any one or more of the four components. Of course, these four components are intrinsically linked and planned change in one area of the organization can sometimes be expected to result in compensatory retaliatory 'unplanned' change in other parts of the system, unless these reactions to change are themselves anticipated and planned for.

Understanding the causes, effects and timescales of these dynamics enables a skilled manager indirectly to influence politically 'sensitive' key sub-systems by ostensibly tackling other apparently unrelated organizational aspects as the focus for change. For example a general manager may target the development of a new operating-theatre regime in order to involve and introduce medical staff to the issues of clinical management within limited resources. Using one focus of manifest change as a vehicle to introduce a related but 'hidden' change of often greater priority is a tried and tested strategy. The extent to which such an approach is successful depends to a large extent on how well the organizational dynamics are understood by the manager initiating change. In Leavitt's words these indirect approaches to change are dependent upon a variety of

> ... assumed casual chains by which they are supposed to bring about their intended changes. Some of the structural approaches, for example, are not aimed directly at tasks but at people as mediating intervening variables. In these approaches, one changes structure to change people to improve task performance. Similarly, some of the people approaches seek to change people in order to change structure and tools, to change task performance, and also to make life more fulfilling for people.

Most efforts to implement programmes of change start from some particular point of origin, but sooner or later must take on board the other types of organizational factors which are always intrinsically linked to the initial point of attack. The sorts of organizational variables and their relative weights and inter-relationships form part of a general manager's mental model of the organization. This understanding of the structure and dynamics of the organization guides the managers' behaviour at all stages of his planned attempts to implement organisational changes. In other words, what managers think about their organizations guides them in what they do about their organizations.

The question of what managers actually do (as discussed in Chapter 2) has occupied a central position within management studies for many years. One descriptive model has traditionally held great sway, although in recent years, many of the assumptions of this 'scientific–rational' approach to management have come increasingly into question. In broad terms, this 'classical' textbook approach sees managerial work as consisting of a number of related activities such as setting objectives, planning, organizing and communicating. Typically, these activities are considered to be regulated by an activity called 'monitoring', which is seen as a means of providing feedback-driven control of the outcomes of the other activities in the set.

Despite its intuitive appeal, this neat structure has not been revealed in observational studies of what managers actually do in their jobs. Two American researchers, Mintzberg (1973) and Kotter (1982), have become clearly identified with a very different alternative to the 'scientific–rational' approach to management. Mintzberg (1975), for example, has stated: 'If you ask a manager what he does he will most likely tell you he plans, organizes, co-ordinates and controls. Then watch what he does. Don't be surprised if you can't relate what you see to these four words.'

As we have seen in Chapter 2, these investigations have revealed that managerial behaviour does not conform to the neatly-demarcated functional activities of the 'classical' approach. In contrast, we are presented with a picture of frantic managerial 'fixing' where little time is spent on any activity in particular, and a great deal of time is spent in brief fragmented conversations with others both inside and outside the organization. Despite the apparent chaotic disorder on the surface, what we are witnessing is, in fact, a systematic and effective means of accumulating a large volume of relevant information coupled with bargaining and bartering for reciprocal 'good turns'. The effective general manager is able to exercise his control and influence over others through brief bursts of purposeful conversation because, as Kotter (1982) has described, his personal agenda for action and his communication networks are very well organized.

Dimmock (1985) has discussed the implications of Kotter's work for the general manager in the NHS, and has pointed out that Kotter's conclusions about what activities make a general manager effective are not in accord with the prevailing NHS view of management. This traditional view sees management as comprising clearly delineated functions such as policy-making, planning, programming and execution.

Consequently, Dimmock contends that the temptation for the newly-appointed general managers to revert to the old established work-patterns will be high unless

1. Health Authorities have clearly specified their organizational objectives and priorities which can form the basis for the general manager's agenda.
2. The general manager can effectively develop a large network of relationships for informational exchange.
3. The general manager has the skill and bargaining acumen effectively to negotiate the thorny issue of resource allocation with the powerful clinical groups.

The application of earlier research findings to the NHS context in this way is useful, but not without some difficulties. The three areas which Dimmock has identified are all necessary but are clearly not sufficient for effective general management. There is a more fundamental factor which cuts across all three areas and which, if absent, has the greatest potential for constraining managers in their attempts to establish new patterns of work in the NHS. Above all else general managers need a clear image of what they intend to achieve and how they intend to get there. They need an appropriate internal mental model of change.

The internal model of change

We have suggested that the hallmark of effective management is the ability to identify, define and structure what managers see as the key features of their organization together with a dynamic model of how these interrelated features are expected to change as a function of their interventions.

Managers need a mental model which enables them to visualize both these structural and process relationships. Achieving this sophisticated level of internal representation is partly a result of a complex and often uncertain process of integrating their experiential learning. Since organizations are always in the process of change and objectively abstracting central features of interest is difficult, the process of experiential learning is bound to be, at best, slow and imperfect, and at worst can lead to serious distortions. Because of the uncertainty of the learning process, general managers often would like to draw upon a body of theoretical knowledge in order to assist them in the development of an appropriate organizational model.

Unfortunately, there are many ways in which organizational change can be conceptualized and, as we have seen in the previous chapter, there is a vast literature which impinges on how change may be understood, predicted and implemented. A general manager searching for the 'best' model of organizational change will be forced to evaluate the relevance of a wide variety of approaches. As we have seen in Chapter 4 these models of change include those which stress organizational inertia, those which stress organizational development, those which focus upon the planning of change, those which describe incremental and integrationship approaches and those which offer prescriptions for the achievement of excellence.

In supporting their theoretical and practical perspectives on the nature and management of organizational change writers on the subject have used a wide range of constructs. The following list illustrates some of the more frequently used dimensions with which these issues have been debated. These dimensions can be broadly categorized as those that refer to types of organizational change and those that refer to the process and management of change.

Types of change

1. Inventive/planned change v. reactive/unplanned change
2. Small-scale change v. large-scale change
3. Radical change v. incremental change
4. Heterogeneous change v. homogeneous change
5. Slow change v. fast change
6. Individual change v. group change
7. Process change v. structural change
8. Strategic change v. cultural change
9. Strategic change v. structural change
10. Attitude/value change v. behaviour/skill change
11. Change as an episode v. change as a sequence of episodes

Process and management of change

12. Intended change outcomes v. unintended change outcomes
13. External triggers to change v. internal triggers to change
14. External change diagnosis v. internal change diagnosis
15. External change agents v. internal change agents
16. Change through transmission v. change through transformation
17. Change by co-operation v. change by conflict

18. Transactional leadership v. transformational leadership
19. Top-down approach v. bottom-up approach
20. Technical problem-solving v. human resource management
21. Behavioural approach v. business strategy approach
22. Reactive management v. proactive management
23. Rational approach v. political approach
24. New vision v. forward planning
25. 'Soft' people skills v. 'hard' quantitative skills
26. Responsiveness to change v. resistance to change
27. Entrepreneurial management v. bureaucratic management
28. Value/culture management v. performance management
29. Change caused by tension v. change caused by choice
30. Creative destruction v. 'unfreezing'
31. Hegemonic control v. negotiated order
32. Change as planning outcome v. change as power struggles outcome
33. Organizational inertia v. organizational momentum
34. Inherited options v. planned interventions

The models which are presented in the literature should be approached with some caution by the practising manager since they often contain contradictory and conflicting evidence and advice. For example, a useful distinction was drawn by Miles (1966) who contrasted the 'human relations model' (in the tradition of Elton Mayo and his followers) with the 'human resources model'. The human relations model is geared toward making people 'feel' more important and the techniques used to increase job satisfaction are seen to be the causes of heightened job performance. On the other hand, the aim of the human resources model is to maximize the use of people's untapped resources and consequently to improve the quality of their work and their job satisfaction. The pivotal difference between the two approaches is the role of job satisfaction, which can be seen either as a cause of or as an effect of heightened job performance.

Work within both these traditions has generated a number of interesting ideas and contrasting the human relation and human resource approaches to work quality and satisfaction becomes more than of passing theoretical interest if we attempt to relate what is implied by these models to the change intervention strategies which a NHS manager might consider attempting when faced with an organizational problem to solve.

As an example, consider a general manager who has ascertained that nursing morale is particularly low on one of his admissions wards. He has also ascertained that absenteeism and number of complaints is high on this ward and suspects, through discussion with nursing staff, that job performance is poor. As an objective he aims to improve both job satisfaction and performance and is considering the alternative strategies he might adopt in achieving this goal. Clearly, if the manager believes that heightened job satisfaction is an important causal factor resulting in increased job performance he is likely to adopt a different sort of approach than if he believes that increased job satisfaction is an effect of improved job performance. In other words, the intervention strategy he chooses to adopt directly depends on his mental model of the situation.

This understanding of the structure and process of the organization enables the skilled manager to judge how he expects the organization to respond to various initiatives and is what is meant when we refer to an internal 'mental model' of an organization. In other words this mental model is some form of internal representation which highlights how salient features of the organization and those internal and external factors which affect them are related to one another. The model is itself dynamic and evolves as a function of training, experience and insight. In a sense, the model is a conceptual framework which includes those constructs which a manager sees as being of central importance in the organization and what factors in the internal and external environment he considers to be potential threats or potential opportunities. The organization is viewed through this conceptual framework and consequently the manager understands which aspects of the organization demand his managerial attention. The nature of the internal mental model guides the way in which managers decide to tackle change. Understanding general managers' strategies and tactics of implementing change firmly rests on understanding how managers themselves understand their organization.

The sorts of models which are used in shaping programmes of change is critical to the success of the general management experiment within the NHS. For those general managers appointed from within the service, the experiential learning on which these models of change are based have been founded in the traditional NHS culture of policy maintenance rather than policy change. For those who have joined the service from other organizations, the degree of transfer of the models of change might be less than they had anticipated. Consequently, all general managers face the problem of changing the culture of their organization whilst simultaneously providing opportunities for all personnel, not least themselves, to acquire rapidly and to internalize useful and shared working models of the emerging organization. If this is to prove successful then they will need to understand and harness the capability of their organizations in order to facilitate this transition effectively.

Formal models and working models

Any attempt to understand the causes, processes and consequences of planned organizational change cannot get very far until we examine the models and motives of the change-agents involved. The general manager is typically faced with difficult questions about the potential risks, benefits and timescale of any approach to change he or she might adopt, and in answering these questions, needs to draw upon his or her internal model of how the organization works. Since general managers are typically faced with very difficult resource allocation problems, and planned programmes of change often need to be justified as 'spend money to save money' exercises, it is imperative that they appreciate not only the immediate consequences of their change attempts, but also the second and third order consequences of their intended strategies. Formal models of the structure of organizations and the processes of organizational change attempt to supply to managers 'off-the-peg' cognitive maps. Having integrated all or part of these approaches, the manager is assumed to have a better 'working' model of his own organization. Unfortunately, off-the-peg models are not always the best fit and occasionally have been made for another customer.

'Models' of organizations are erected as practical frameworks for management and have typically partitioned organizations into components or 'elements' as a means of providing a conceptual framework for assessing current functioning and effectiveness. Kotter (1978), for example, presents a model which comprises the following seven major elements.

1. Key organizational processes
2. The external environment
3. Employees and other tangible assets
4. Formal organizational arrangements
5. The internal social system
6. The organization's technology
7. The dominant coalition.

Similarly, Harrison (1987) presents an 'open-systems' model which comprises the following eight main elements.

1. Input or resources
2. Outputs
3. Technology
4. Environment (task and general)
5. Purposes (strategies and plans)
6. Behaviour and processes
7. Culture
8. Structure

There are, of course, many more examples of similar analysis schemes scattered throughout the literature. These two are included as up-to-date examples.

Despite the surface semantic differences between these two lists of organizational components, intuitively there seems to be a great deal of overlap between the two. For example, Kotter's internal social system seems broadly equivalent to Harrison's culture component; Kotter's formal organizational arrangement is akin to Harrison's structure component and so on. In a similar way the list of differing models and components proposed by different authors could be extended almost indefinitely. In almost every case the components would have been selected on some or all of the following criteria. These criteria are perfectly sensible and typically comprise importance or relevance, mutual exclusivity, exhaustivity, and usefulness. Use of criteria typically ensures the internal validity of the proposed model. Unfortunately despite the internal integrity of most of these models, there is little external integrity since it is never a clear-cut matter to compare any one model with another. When different models are examined, it is not always apparent whether or not similar terms refer to similar aspects of the organization and conversely, whether different terms refer to similar organizational features. This example is included to illustrate the problem of imprecision in the welter of terms, concepts and constructs used to describe organizations. Making meaningful comparisons across different theories and models is often fraught because of the confusing and idiosyncratic use of jargon.

However, despite this confusion, models of this sort can prove useful in several ways. Firstly, they can be used as aids in the diagnosis of organizational state since each of the components may be related to sets of questions which focus thinking on relevant organizational information. For example, both Kotter and Harrison (like many others) provide lists of questions for each of their model components. Attempting to answer these questions, however imperfectly, means that managers are prompted to consider a wide range of those organizational factors which are likely to impact upon their decision-making.

The second use of models is that they suggest how the organizational components or variables tend to interact. The relationships between these elements can be analyzed for a particular organizational scenario and appropriate 'working' models of the organization can be derived. As we have discussed earlier, if design and change are to take place in a systematic manner then general managers (and everyone else involved) require a clear model or cognitive map which shows how one step follows from another in moving toward the goal of a particular change.

A key part of any model then is the specification of these relationships. Ideally, the model should outline the complete set of cause and effect relationships between its components, but often this level of specification cannot be fully accomplished because we simply do not know the ways in which many important organizational components interrelate. Consequently, other less powerful relationships which more realistically represent our state of knowledge of organizational functioning are sometimes included. In these cases it is not possible confidently to state that one factor causes another; instead the most that can be claimed is that one factor affects another.

The causal relationships

There is a huge variety of causal relationships which have been implicitly or explicitly stated in the literature on organizational change. Many of these have been touched upon in Chapter 4, and often resemble simple 'if then' rules when examined in isolation. For example the literature suggests (along with a multitude of other cause–effect relationships)

If employees have negative attitudes **then** there tends to be conflict and inefficiency.
If organizations are highly bureaucratic **then** there tends to be less organizational creativity.
If environmental changes are not predictable **then** this tends to result in less long-term planning.
And so on.

These 'rules' or causal relationships can be listed, compared and contrasted in a variety of permutations. In many ways these 'rules' resemble proverbs. Like proverbs, they reside in the realm of 'common sense' and often go unchallenged or unquestioned. Like proverbs, completely contradictory 'rules' can often be found. To take an example discussed earlier 'job dissatisfaction causes poor work performance' and 'poor work performance causes job dissatisfaction'. In a similar way the direction of the cause–effect relationship between organizational strategy and structure has been extensively debated without resolution.

One of the main problems with thinking and reasoning about real organizations is that the causal relationships which constitute the 'expert' body of knowledge on organizational dynamics are often statements of belief rather than statements of knowledge. Whereas logic assumes that facts are statements which always remain true, in the reality of organizational life 'facts' have a tendency to change their status as true or false as evidence accumulates over time. Coupled with the additional issue that it is much more usual for organizational 'facts' not to be simply perceived as being either true or false but rather as relatively likely or unlikely, it is clear that organizational facts are vaguer and more changeable than the polarities of traditional logic can cater for.

There have been numerous attempts to extend the traditional two-valued (i.e. true or false) logics to cope better with the more flexible ways in which people actually think about real issues. One approach (the so-called non-monotonic logics) has been to devise systems of logic which can embrace the problem of 'facts' changing their status from true to false or vice versa as evidence accumulates. The other approach has been to abandon the traditional restriction that facts can only assume the two values of true and false. In this approach (the multi-valued logics) facts are not categorized as simply true or false; instead they are allowed to assume a range of values and meanings between these two extremes. In a three-valued logic, statements may be classified as true, false or undecided; the last category is a pending category which awaits further evidence. Four-, five- and six-valued logics have been proposed for particular situations, and the utility of these logics rests upon the interpretation of the truth values for each category.

It seems then that the truth of organizational statements often lies somewhere between the extremes of true and false. This situation occurs because of the lack of precision in the way in which organizational concepts are used and described.

Traditional logic assumes that it is possible to say whether a statement is true or false and if we represent true by 1 and false by 0 then all statements can be assigned one or other of these two values. On the other hand, one type of multi-valued logic, fuzzy logic allows an infinite number of truth values between these extremes of 1 and 0. For example, if we take the statement, 'Some surgeons work quicker than others' then traditional logic would suggest that the statement 'Surgeon X works quickly' can be deemed to be true or false. However, it is clear that the term 'quicker' is not precisely defined. If a general manager examined the performance of surgeons, he might be prepared to say that twenty operations a week is quick and even nineteen operations a week is quick but five operations a week is slow. What about the case of ten operations performed per week? In a sense the general manager might say that the statement 'Surgeon Y performs ten operations per week' is only 0.5 true. In this way fuzzy logic can cope with degrees of truth.

As in traditional logic, fuzzy logic propositions can be joined together into larger rule statements. For example, a general manager may be using rules of the following type.

If 'Surgeon X works quickly' **and** 'Y resources are available' **then** 'waiting-list gets smaller'.

If 'Surgeon X works quickly' **or** Surgeon Y works quickly' **then** 'Resources deplete faster'.

Since the 'rules' which managers use are rarely universally applicable and are based upon their particular belief systems, it can be extremely misleading to consider a simplistic linking of organizational components without taking into account the wider context of all the other components of the system. For example, Kotter (1978) has stated: 'I have seen dozens of examples . . . in which managers or organization specialists misdiagnosed what was causing some type of short-run dynamic because they implicitly were using an inadequate model of the situation.'

If we are to understand the processes by which a general manager implements change, we need to understand how he or she perceives the organization and how it is considered to develop under his or her management. In other words, we need to appreciate how the general manager's working model of the system anticipates and traces the sequence of organizational stages and transitions.

Ultimately, we are interested in examining the effectiveness of any general manager's change interventions. The question of time-scale is of importance here. The short-term nature of most general managers' contracts of employment means that if they are to achieve realistic change then they need to achieve these innovations within a relatively short time-scale.

Unfortunately, it is very easy to underestimate the amount of time and effort required to achieve signficant organizational change. Coupled with this issue is the added complexity that the dynamics which characterize short-term organizational dynamics are often not the same as those which characterize long-term organizational dynamics. Consequently, utilizing a strategy of maintaining general managers on short-term contracts may well result in quite different change initiatives than would be the case if they were employed on a longer-term basis. The next section describes the types of organizational change programmes which general managers are attempting to implement.

The programmes of change

The NHS is a large and complex system organized to meet the varied health needs of the community. Despite its enormity of scale and diversity of health care objectives, it is essentially one unified human system. The practice of general management in the NHS requires a sensitive and skilled handling of this human dimension which must be recognized as of fundamental importance in shaping both the content and approach of managerial work in the health care arena. The work of general managers is, above all, to manage human systems. Within this ever-changing milieu of interacting care providers and clients, general managers are expected to champion the new ethos of 'managerialism'. The primary role of the general manager is to spearhead the transition of the NHS from a passive administration and maintenance culture to an active and innovatory management culture geared to positive organizational intervention.

The breadth of on-going and proposed changes will entail the emergence of new managerial structures, new systems and procedures, and new policies and programmes. Despite the medical profession's concerns with what they see as 'unwise haste', these innovations are considered by many to require rapid implementation at all levels in the NHS if they are to prove successful. The introduction of general management is largely synonymous with encouraging, planning and implementing a wide range of organizational changes and these changes may encompass not only major large-scale system design and redesign but also minor fine-tuning of organizational functioning on a daily basis.

The breadth of changes with which a general manager is concerned may range from encouraging clinicians to participate in the management process, attacking long waiting lists, estate management ventures, performance appraisal or the development of incentives for staff. The programmes of change are many and varied and were precipitated as a direct result of the Griffiths proposals.

The Griffiths Report was not intended to be a cost-cutting exercise, a manpower enquiry or simply another scheme for reorganization of the NHS. Rather it was directed toward making recommendations about effective management of the NHS. As we have seen, Griffiths argued that there was too much centralized control, decision-making was too ponderous, and consensus management was resulting in widespread organizational inertia. These identified problems needed tackling through a more rigorous and accountable management structure, and the impact of these changes is now cascading through the region, district and unit levels of the service.

In order to examine current programmes of change, we asked a sample of 55 general managers to list those specific changes that are or will be taking place in their units or districts in the foreseeable future. A total of 251 organizational changes were identified by the general managers in the sample and these were coded into ten categories which are shown with their respected frequencies, percentage frequencies and ranks in table 5.1. For the majority of changes included in table 5.1, general managers were both personally committed to and often personally involved in their practical implementation.

The ten types of critical change included in table 5.1 can be broadly partitioned into two groups. The most frequently cited change categories are A and B which represent two inclusive category groups which can encompass the remaining eight categories (C–J) to a varying extent. Broadly, we found that general managers have two overall priorities for change. The first can be called 'substantive' priorities and these are concerned with types of changes related to assessing and restructuring provisions and services. The second broad class of change can be called 'symbolic' priorities and these are directed toward engendering acceptance of the new general management ethos and culture. For example, decentralizing services from a main hospital into the community (Category A – substantive change) may entail changing methods of budgeting and financial control (Category F change) together with a restructuring of managerial responsibilities (Category C change).

On the other hand, attempting to create a more positive cultural climate (Category B – symbolic change) could also involve redefining the clinicians' role in management (Category G change) and delegating responsibility (Category D change). Clearly the categories of critical changes rarely occur in isolation and are interrelated in many ways. Examining general managers' priorities for change through a series of case studies has highlighted that both substantive and symbolic change need to go hand-in-hand if innovation is to be successful. These case studies and the managerial strategies behind their implementation are discussed in Chapter 8.

Table 5.1 Frequency and rank of critical organizational changes for 55 general managers

	Category of key change	Frequency of critical changes	% Frequency	Rank
A	Assessing and restructuring provisions and services	61	24.3	1
B	Engendering acceptance of new management attitudes, ethos and culture	47	18.7	2
C	Changing management structure	26	10.4	3
D	Delegating responsibility and ensuring accountability	25	10.0	4
E	Performance appraisal	22	8.8	5
F	Changing methods of budgeting and financial control	19	7.6	6
G	Redefining the medical role in management	17	6.8	7
H	Changing methods of strategic management and planning	15	6.0	8
I	Improving communication and information	13	5.2	9
J	Ensuring appropriate staff development and training	6	2.4	10

The results revealed an interesting pattern in the general managers' change priorities. Categories C and E, changing management structure and performance appraisal are often linked to either the substantive Category A or the symbolic Category B. However, the 'task-orientated' change categories H and F (changing methods of strategic management and planning and changing methods of budgeting and financial control) are more likely to be associated with Category A than Category B. Conversely, the 'people-orientated' change categories D and I (delegating responsibility and ensuring accountability and improving communication and information) are more likely to be associated with Category B than Category A. Categories G and J (redefining the medical role in management and ensuring appropriate staff development and training) are both approximately equally likely to be associated with either Category A or Category B.

These results demonstrate that general managers clearly recognize the importance of attempting to engender both symbolic and substantive change, although there were clear differences in general managers' inclination to use either symbolic or substantive changes as their initial targets for attack. As the impact of these changes unfold, there is a heightened awareness that justification of these changes must eventually be evaluated on the basis of improved health care delivery to the patients, although at this early stage in the general management experiment it is not always possible to evaluate the long-term care outcomes of change.

In instigating these innovations, many would contend that the success of a general manager will ultimately rest on his ability to shape actively the ideas of all the people who work in his part of the NHS. From this perspective, the primary role of the general manager is, in Zaleznik's (1977) words, 'to change the way people think about what is desirable, possible and necessary'. In other words, many believe that person-orientated symbolic change lies at the heart of the effective management of innovation.

In a similar vein, it has been frequently contended that changing the organizational structure and culture of the NHS requires that the general manager provides a clear unified 'vision' of the organizational goals and purposes whilst striving to inculcate the new beliefs and values which are required to support and facilitate the new initiatives for change. To this end, leadership that goes beyond merely managing the work that others do appears to be a prerequisite for success, but exactly what this implies for a general manager in terms of his or her perceptions, attitudes and behaviour is a complex issue. The definition and measurement of the 'effectiveness' of a general manager in implementing change can be tackled in a number of ways, and some of these approaches are considered in later chapters.

What is apparent is that understanding how managers bring about change cannot be fully tackled merely by considering what managers do. In order to understand the process of change we must know how the general manager views the change process and the goals, values and expectations on which this process is founded. Therefore, in this early phase of general management it is especially important to understand how general managers view the direction in which the organization is currently travelling and if, how and why they intend to change course.

Harnessing organizational capability

The examination of current programmes of change has highlighted the importance of both substantive and symbolic change strategies in the repertoire of general mangers. These programmes will require general mangers to harness effectively the skills and experience of those in their organizations to develop and maintain shared objectives of change.

The NHS is a large sprawling organization composed of a huge number of roles, many of which have evolved slowly and which are perpetuated by traditional work practices and procedures. In the past these traditional roles have been a stabilizing force and even in these turbulent times can be expected to provide some useful degree of continuity with the past.

Unfortunately, the momentum of the past can sometimes prove too powerful and this often mitigates against attempts to change radically the way the organization functions. Under the aegis of general management innovations are being enthusiastically pursued and many of these changes are occurring both because of and in spite of the relative scarcity of economic and human resources. The organizational pressure that flows from this under-resourcing heightens the perceived necessity for change, and despite resistance, general managers are keen to improve the efficiency and effectiveness of the districts, regions and units which they control. If it can be harnessed effectively, this enthusiasm may prove of great value in their mission to bring about the transformation of the NHS.

Within the NHS there is a wealth and diversity of existing knowledge, skills and expertise across many domains and located at all levels of the service. In their attempt to facilitate the transition from the old reactive rule-based behaviour to a more dynamic stance, general managers as the key agents of organizational change will need to harness existing resources, skills and expertise much more effectively than they have previously been utilized.

The view that people at work are often underutilized, not merely in terms of work effort but also in their potential for exercising responsibility, creativity and leadership has often been voiced. However, improving the utilization of organizational capability has received scant examination from those studying the nature and application of skills in organizations. As Heller (1971) has pointed out, occupational psychologists have typically concentrated their attention on two main areas. These are, firstly, the identification of existing skills via the fields of testing and selection, and secondly, the creation of new skills through the techniques of training and development. Consequently there is a dearth of useful information relating to either the theory or practice of utilizing the wide range of available skills lying untapped throughout an organization. Despite this neglect from researchers there is an increasing realization that organizations have a value beyond their economic worth and this has become increasingly recognized and captured in such phrases as 'human resource' or 'human asset' accounting. This wider view of organizational worth naturally leads to a consideration of how untapped and unexploited human skills and abilities can be better utilized in serving the organization's goals. These human resource aspects of the organization have traditionally been the concern of the personnel function but the potential value of this untapped reservoir of knowledge, skills and abilities has been increasingly recognized by senior management.

The human resource perspective

Successfully managing people at work is the business of all managers at all levels in any organization but this is particularly the case for human service organizations. Many general managers have recognized this need and have appointed specialized personnel staff who have been specifically charged with the responsibility of initiating, implementing and monitoring personnel policies in a wide range of manpower areas. Typically, personnel specialists deal with such organizational activities as recruitment, training, management development, reward structures and redundancy. The concern of many general managers is to evaluate the worth of these activities for their staff in developing manpower policy. However, in examining the issue of the value of the human side of their enterprise many general managers have called into question those who might have been expected to provide some of the answers.

The cost-effectiveness of specialist personnel work itself and the organizational value of this work has been increasingly scrutinized. The main source of criticism has emanated from those managers who have suggested, sometimes unfairly, that there is no demonstrable link between personnel policies and organizational efficiency. In some sectors of the NHS specialist personnel activities are already viewed as 'icing on the cake', expensive and not strictly necessary for survival. However, effective general managers must be concerned with quantifying the effects of their management strategies upon the cost and value of people as an organizational resource. Consequently, they need to understand the effects of their decisions on the human part of the organization and assess the consequences, costs and benefits of their strategic plans.

In developing manpower policy, a general manager needs to take account of the distinction between the effectiveness and the efficiency of such policies. Whereas effectiveness is concerned with the extent to which policies support and facilitate the wider objectives of the organization, efficiency is concerned with the costs of delivering any particular policy. Assessing effectiveness is problematic since organizational objectives are often not specified in sufficient detail and even those strategic objectives which are clearly stated are subject to rapid change as circumstances alter.

Assessing efficiency must entail the continuous monitoring of manpower policies in order that their relevance and impact can be evaluated and this activity itself requires time and money.

These practical hurdles to assessment coupled with general management's lack of faith in the cash value of many traditional personnel techniques has frequently resulted in a reluctance to commit resources to monitor the cost benefits of personnel policies. However, as general management's awareness of the scale of employment costs grows this may change, although many believe that continuing lack of assessment together with the absence of adequate techniques for measuring the efficiency of personnel policies has been largely responsible for the decline in status and influence of many personnel specialists. However, the traditional role of the personnel specialist has been reconceptualized in many successful businesses so that their responsibility has moved from designing and implementing particular policies, to providing advice about the human resource implications of management strategy. Despite the disillusion in some quarters with the techniques and methods which personnel specialists use, there is widespread agreement that it is vital to assess the human resource implications of a broad spectrum of management decisions and strategies. General managers need to understand the long-range consequences and hidden costs of their organizational interventions.

Cost-benefit analysis

Cost-benefit analysis is a way of demonstrating the costs and benefits of policies so that rational decisions can be made about how policies may be adapted or amended in the light of this information. This rational approach to decision-making is fine in theory but there are a number of practical reasons why it is so rarely utilized in practice. Some of these are briefly noted below.

– There is a wide range of costs and these can be historical, replacement or opportunity costs. Deciding which are appropriate in a particular situation is problematic.
– Deciding on the time-scale over which the benefits are to be assessed can prove difficult in practice.
– It is impossible to catalogue completely all costs, and although historical costs can be identified, replacement costs provide a more accurate basis for decision-making particularly in times of high inflation. The measurement of opportunity costs is always hypothetical.
– Finding a costing procedure that is valid for all manpower decisions is extremely difficult but without similar procedures it becomes impossible to evaluate the different manpower policies.
– The data required to perform cost-benefit analyses are often inaccessible or too expensive to obtain.
– Often there appears to be no quantifiable 'objective' benefit for many manpower policies.

Clearly, the full cost of inadequate selection decisions is much greater than the money spent on recruitment, training and wages, Good employees are far more productive than bad ones but calculating the value of any particular worker is extremely difficult in practice. This is particularly true for complex jobs where there is no clear-cut measure of output, and for these jobs the accepted wisdom has been that it is impossible to calculate directly the cash value of an employee.

Recently, however, techniques have been devised to put a cash value on any worker doing any job no matter how complex and intangible. The 'rational estimate' technique relies on a number of supervisors judging the employee's worth and despite criticism of the subjectivity of the approach, there is some evidence to demonstrate its validity. Estimates have been used to calculate the savings made by using effective selection methods and may have a wider application as useful criteria in other cost-benefit analyses of manpower functions.

Evaluating the cash benefits of manpower policies implies the availability of quantitative auditing techniques which are both reliable and valid. Unfortunately it is not always possible to quantify directly the effects of these policies in cost-benefit terms, although well-structured activities such as recruitment and training are better suited to quantitative analysis than other more nebulous activities like providing advice or improving communications. In some instances it is difficult to determine or even estimate costs or benefits although often it is these ill-defined activities which are generally perceived as contributing the most to productivity. In other instances, it is impossible to determine accurately the return on expenditure although the costs of various approaches can be ascertained. For these situations, a cost-minimization strategy may be adopted whereby the cheapest solution is sought for a given amount of output or activity.

Despite these reservations, a number of quantitative techniques may be used to infer the success or otherwise of manpower policies, but any approach that is adopted requires access to appropriate data. Frequently, the accounting conventions in an organization do not provide data which are broken down into categories of employment costs and consequently it is necessary to adapt the existing accounting techniques if personnel cost assessment is to proceed. The benefits of costing manpower policies can be substantial since without measures of policy performance it is impossible to manipulate policies effectively. Unfortunately, obtaining satisfactory measures of the results of manpower policies is not a simple matter and much debate surrounds the use of various measures and approaches.

Perhaps the real problem with cost-benefit analysis is that the decision-making of senior management does not take place using a rational process of comparing the relative values of different strategic approaches. In reality, the micro-politics of the organization remain the real driving force behind the managers' tactics and strategies, although establishing the monetary costs and benefits of manpower policies is generally useful even if subsequent decision-making is driven more by subjective than objective judgement.

Human resource accounting (HRA)

The purpose of human resource accounting is to help management use an organization's human resources more efficiently and effectively. The previous discussion of cost-benefit analysis has highlighted that the fundamental problem with this approach is that the quality and quantity of information necessary to apply the technique are typically not available.

The general manager requires various types of information to manage the human resources of an organization and from this perspective the primary role of human resource accounting is to provide this information. Consequently, human resource accounting systems generally start from identifying the type of information needed to manage the organization's human resources effectively.

In order to obtain this information, it is necessary to quantify the costs and value of people in the organization and it is fundamental to the approach that employees are seen as assets, not just as costs. Consequently, factors such as education, training, and employment costs represent investments in people which should be measurable. There is a diversity of ways in which these investments can be measured, ranging from fairly simplistic human asset balances based on acquisition costs and employees' expected working life to more complex methods which attempt to incorporate psychological measures of satisfaction, motivation and effort.

Human resource accounting can, in theory, provide a conceptual framework and a range of techniques to provide management with 'hard' numerical information which can be used to optimize management decision-making. Unfortunately, in practice attempting to measure people as assets is a difficult procedure. These difficulties stem from two main sources. Firstly there is some theoretical confusion with respect to a number of the concepts used. Secondly, it is not always appropriate to transfer accounting conventions to humans. Human assets, unlike more conventional assets, are outside the direct control of management.

Human resource accounting has not lived up to the expectations of its early proponents but does have value as a conceptual framework in which to provide the general manager with the information needed to apply the techniques of cost-benefit analysis to the evaluation of manpower policies. Its methods and theory are still in the process of development but there is recently a renewed interest in its development and this may lead to a clarification of some of its assumptions.

Performance indicators

Whereas cost-benefit analysis and human resource accounting are complex approaches to the issues of assessing the value of manpower, many organizations make use of much simpler performance indicators which relate employment costs to productivity. These indicators include employee-based ratios such as profit per employee, costs per employee, capital per employee etc., and employment cost percentages such as employment costs as a percentage of profit, employment costs as a percentage of cash flow, etc. These measures have the advantage of simplicity and in certain instances can prove useful to management as rough and ready indicators of organizational performance.

In the NHS such performance indicators include manpower indicators such as beds per consultant, discharges per consultant, consultants per 100 000 population and so on; workload indicators such as length of stay, turnover interval, available beds per 1000 catchment population amongst others, and other district and hospital-based indicators relating to such factors as waiting lists, discharges, deaths and throughput.

The Korner Steering Group on Health Service Information recommended that a common basic set of data should be collected by all health authorities and this has been proceeding since April 1987. This data is intended to be relevant to the local management of health services and is being used as the basis for the development of a package of performance indicators by a national advisory group. In a recent paper on performance indicators in the NHS management process, Harley (1988) has discussed the scope of such approaches and highlighted some important practical issues for their use by general managers. Harley points out that the use of performance indicators is established within the NHS, but general managers are reluctant to use them. This lack of enthusiasm is attributed to the fact that although there is a great deal of information about resource inputs and the processes of care, there is little corresponding information about the outcomes of health care. Without this outcome information the evaluation of performance is seen as tenuous and unstable. However, whilst recognising that the data is imperfect, Harley argues that performance indicators do reveal valid comparative information between hospitals and districts. In fact, comparative data of this type is used extensively by central and regional authorities in their performance and accountability reviews.

However, many managers and clinicians still believe that these performance indicators tend to be too gross as measures to enable the performance of different hospitals and districts to be effectively assessed. They feel that organizational performance is influenced by a whole range of factors which cannot be captured by such crude measures. Measuring performance at work is a complicated issue since individuals, jobs and organizational expectations vary such a great deal between contexts. Consequently, performance indicator antagonists consider that productivity often cannot be defined in any simple way which can be universally applied across all health care contexts and therefore cannot be adequately assessed using simple performance indicators.

Whether the information provided by current performance indicators is valid or not, it is widely felt that a shared database which is acceptable to both managers and medics alike could provide a sound foundation on which to base the selection of organizational issues and priorities and provide a means for better planning of services. Unfortunately, however reliable and valid any data is, this data still requires interpretation, and it seems clear that managers and medics have fundamentally different models of the system in which they work. These differences are not trivial and the contrasting values and belief systems of managers and medics are quite likely to result in very different interpretations of the identical agreed database. It may be wishful thinking on the part of management to assume that 'if there is comparative data available national-ly and the data is published every year, then criticism of ones own consultants becomes easier and *has* to be accepted by the clinicians' (Harley, 1988 – our emphasis).

However, it does seem clear that the use of widely accepted performance indicators can have a real impact upon the utilization of manpower within the NHS and this can operate at two distinct levels. Firstly, differing practices between consultants can be exposed and poor performers identified. Secondly, agreed performance indicators could provide the basis for a common model of the health-care system for both managers and clinicians.

Performance indicators themselves could provide the starting point for identifying those components of the system which are seen as important. The ways in which these components are structured and represented in the internal mental models of managers and clinicians could then be examined. It seems reasonable to assume that exposing the implicit causal relationships of different individuals' mental models of a system would further test the reliability and validity of many of the implicit assumptions on which the conflict between managers and medics is based.

CHAPTER 6
Examining working models of change

General managers, like everybody else, have a combination of certain innate and acquired abilities which they use in dealing with their world. The manner in which a general manager thinks or acts with respect to an organizational disturbance is determined by his or her mental representations or 'schemata' for understanding or dealing with the issues at hand. Consequently, it seems reasonable to assume that a manager has a range of schemata for dealing with different sorts of organizational scenarios. The term 'schemata' is often used in a similar way to a range of other terms in the literature. These other terms include 'mental maps', 'cognitive maps', 'frames', 'plans', and 'scripts' amongst others. All of these terms refer to cognitive (i.e. mental) representations of attributes and the relationships between them and so all of these terms refer to 'cognitive structures', another term which is frequently applied to the problem of describing internal mental representations of reality. These terms have been debated by cognitive scientists and various distinctions drawn between them. For example, a 'cognitive map' is sometimes taken to be a part of the broader term, 'schema' and a 'script' appears to be more action-oriented than a 'frame'. In a sense they are all mental maps since they are used in guiding an individual's behaviour in relation to his goals and circumstances.

However, the distinctions between the uses of this variety of terms is currently not completely clear and we generally prefer to use the term 'mental model' to refer to a manager's internal representation of the organization. These mental models can never be fully complete or wholly specified and are always subject to review in the light of experience. To use a previous analogy they are 'working models' of on-going organizational events which need to be broadly correct; if these working models are too incomplete or misleading, then we would expect that the general manager's performance as change agent is likely to be misdirected and inadequate.

The extent to which general managers are employing adequate models of organizational dynamics is critical in assessing the effectiveness of their programmes of change. The role of information in maintaining managers' grasp of current organizational conditions and their relationship with the working models are subsequently described and used to further our understanding of the process of innovation in the NHS. The remainder of this chapter introduces a simple but useful technique for examining general managers' working models of change and uses a case-study to illustrate the steps involved in this sort of analysis. Chapter 7 presents several more case-studies in order to highlight some practical issues in implementing organizational change. Chapters 8 and 9 introduce two further specific research techniques for examining aspects of managers' models of change and describe some issues which these have revealed.

Information and decision-making

The turbulent post-Griffiths climate within the NHS has increased uncertainty and fuelled the demand for information to reduce this uncertainty throughout all levels of the service. If the new breed of general managers is required to make better decisions then they require better information on which to base them.

Those who emphasize information's role as a support to managerial decision-making often consider that, above all other activities, the key task of management is to make decisions under conditions of varying uncertainty. Good information is seen as vital because it reduces this uncertainty, although there are different sorts of managerial decisions only some of which can lead to the specification of the optimal solution. For example, Ackoff (1967) postulated three types of managerial decision characterized by the degree of uncertainty inherent under each. The degree of uncertainty increases as we pass from decision-type (a), through type (b), to type (c).

(a) Decisions for which adequate models are available and from which optimal solutions can be derived.
(b) Decisions from which adequate models can be constructed but from which optimal solutions cannot be derived.
(c) Decisions for which adequate models cannot be constructed.

This typology of managerial decision-making suggests that there are two components in making a decision. Firstly, an adequate model of the decision-space is required and this mental model should contain valid information about the causes and consequences of the factors deemed to be relevant to the decision at hand. Secondly, in addition to an adequate model of the decision situation, the manager needs to be able to derive optimal solutions from an understanding of this model and this production of solutions may occur with varying degrees of success. One way of examining uncertainty and decision-making is the well-known scheme proposed by Thompson and Tuden (1959). These authors distinguish two sorts of uncertainty stemming from the cause-and-effect relationships which are part of how organizational actions and reactions are understood by managers. The suggested relationships between these two types of uncertainty and organizational decision-making is shown below.

| Low uncertainty of cause and effect | Decision by |
| Low uncertainty of objectives | computation |

| Low uncertainty of cause and effect | Decision by |
| High uncertainty of objectives | compromise |

High uncertainty of cause and effect   } Decision by
Low uncertainty of objectives   judgement

High uncertainty of cause and effect   } Decision by
High uncertainty of objectives   inspiration

If organizational objectives are generally agreed and cause–effect relations are clear then it is possible to impose decision-making by computation. At the other extreme, if both objectives and cause–effect relations are contentious then there is only the potential for inspirational decision making. Decision-making by compromise and judgement are indicated when either clarity of causal relations or clarity of objectives are relatively low.

This sort of framework is useful in attempting to understand the manner in which information may support decision-making and relates to another model, 'the information processing perspective', which views an organization in terms of the flow and processing of information. Galbraith is a major proponent of the information processing view of organizations. From this perspective, the greater the uncertainty of the task, the greater the amount of information that has to be processed during the execution of the task. If the task is well understood much of the activity can be pre-planned prior to execution. For example, Galbraith (1974) has stated: 'the greater the task uncertainty, the greater the amount of information that must be processed among decision-makers during task execution in order to achieve a given level of performance'.

The concept of task uncertainty is useful in understanding how tasks, information processing and organizational structure are interrelated. In large complex organizations, it is necessary to partition the organizational tasks among several groups and then to integrate the sub-tasks to accomplish the overall organizational mission. There are a number of strategies which are available when co-ordinating and integrating sub-tasks, and these can range from developing standard operating procedures and decision rules, establishing a hierarchy within which exceptions to the rules can be referred to the next higher level, or setting the goals or targets of each sub-task and delegating the method of accomplishing the goal to the personnel involved in the sub-task. In addition to the strategic responses, a great deal of uncertainty can increase the capacity of the organization to process information by creating new information systems. Consequently, it is important that management should not emphasize the development of any new manual or computer-based information system in isolation from its organizational context.

Although it seems reasonable to assume that information is an essential raw material for decision-making, many managers question the existence of a simple relationship between management information systems and effective organizational performance. The reason for this apparent paradox is that organizations have a number of 'modes' in which information is transmitted and processed. Information may be of a number of types which can be variously described as official or unofficial, routine or non-routine, formal or informal, etc. The unofficial, informal information that managers frequently use in making critical decisions often does not emanate from a formal information system, although the extent to which 'informal' information could or should be encapsulated in an information system is an unresolved issue.

Dearden (1972), for example, has argued that since a computer-based management information system does not include important qualitative information it has little impact on the large non-computer-based information, decision and control systems which are probably far more important for effective management. Grinyer and Norburn (1975) found no significant relationship between formal information systems and financial performance; rather, they found greater management utilization of informal channels of communication and decision-making was associated with success. Similarly, Mintzberg (1972) has demonstrated that top managers prefer and select informal modes of information processing and many others have observed that management appears to thrive in an atmosphere of multiple, informal and re-negotiated exchanges of information.

In many ways information and communication are two sides of the same coin, and if real improvements are to be made in organizational performance, then it will prove necessary for the designers of new information systems to expand their notions of what constitutes 'normal' management. Systems designers, particularly those with a technical data-processing background, frequently hold a number of implicit assumptions about the ways in which managers make decisions. They seem to believe that managers are or aim to be completely objective, logical and fact-orientated and that their decision-making is always rationally planned well in advance of actually implementing any organizational change. In this view subjective 'soft' informal communication is thought to be of little importance to a manager's important decisions and actions. This 'rationality' stereotype is extremely misleading. The narrow focus of the technical approach can only lead to marginal organizational improvements, since it neglects the wider social ramifications of information innovations and even curtails the type of information considered to be useful. Viewing information as an essentially technical phenomena leads to a distorted view of the role of information in organizations and a broader more inclusive outlook is necessary in order to incorporate important informal aspects of information and communication.

Whatever sorts and sources of information best suit the requirements of managers, it is clear that general managers in the NHS are required to make many decisions and these decisions range from the infrequent highest level strategic decision to determine future policy and organizational direction to the more frequent and mundane decisions which are necessary to control the organization on a day-to-day basis. In an attempt to understand the process of decision-making, the activity has often been presented as a series of well-demarcated stages. In these approaches, the behaviour of the decision-maker is traced from the original problem recognition and definition stages through the stages of searching for and selecting alternative solutions to the final stage of implementing the decision in managerial action. The neatness of the sequential stage approach is rarely, if ever, found in real decision-making since both the stages and the sequence of events are never so clear-cut as the model suggests. However, the model does have an intuitive appeal and can prove useful as a framework for viewing some aspects of decision-making for organizational change.

Recognition of the need to initiate change

At the early recognition stage of the change process, it is essential that general managers have the ability to recognize those organizational cues which signal that a problem exists. Those organizational events which alert a manager to the existence of a problem are generally thought to be those which highlight discrepancies between what is and what ought to be. However, these discrepancies are not always immediately apparent and often have to be discovered through the processes controlled by the manager's mental models of the organization. The recogniton of problems depends not only on the organizational events themselves but on the ways in which an individual manager interprets these events. Different general managers have different strategies in allocating time between the maintenance of existing operations and the active search for threats and opportunities, and these individual differences are reflected in their occupational personalities and management styles. However, irrespective of these differences between the temperament and outlook of individual managers, it has been frequently demonstrated that there are a number of essential conditions for the effective recognition of the need to initiate strategies of organizational change. Some of these conditions are personal and therefore related to the individual manager and some of these conditions are related to the structure and culture of the organization.

Individual conditions for facilitating change recognition

Three conditions appear to be particularly relevant for sensitizing the individual general manager to effective recognition of organizational problems. These are ensuring sensitivity to organizational signals, ensuring access to good data, and ensuring the effective interpretation of information.

In a complex and rapidly changing environment like the NHS, there are many cues, clues and signals which may herald potential problems and these are incessantly presenting themselves for further attention. It is essential that managers ensure that all of these are not given the same priority since the management systems would quickly become overloaded and ineffectual. Managers need to be selective to those situations which they choose to act on but it is in this act of selective filtering that there are two potential sources of danger. Firstly, over-controlling problem recognition results in an over-passive management style. Secondly, selecting the wrong organizational issues for further consideration can prove at best inconvenient and at worst potentially disastrous. Clearly it is important that general managers are active and action-oriented since an over-complacent approach is incompatible with their key role as agents of change. The potential problem of an over-passive management style is primarily tackled by ensuring that active managers are selected to fill these critical organizational roles. The second potential danger is more complex.

It seems that a crucial difference between an effective and an ineffective general manager lies in the ability to predict which organizational events are good or bad predictors of future organizational situations. This ability depends not only upon formal organizational procedures and control mechanisms which are specifically designed to reduce managerial uncertainty but also upon informal signals from inside and outside the organization. We have seen that building and maintaining a contact network is a critical activity for successful general management, and it is through these contacts that the effective manager gets a 'feel' for who and what is worth listening to. The effective general manager needs to ensure that he has adequate access to both 'hard' factual data and 'soft' impressionistic data.

It must be remembered that merely collecting this data is not enough, since data needs to be converted into information to be useful and in turn this information needs to be appropriately interpreted. It is important to stress that the general manager does not passively absorb the data which he receives through written reports or through his own experiences. Events or situations can never be fully described objectively since these organizational stimuli are always subject to an individual manager's interpretation. A manager attaches meaning to each organizational situation in accordance with his own experiences, attitudes and values. In other words, his mental model shapes his perception of the situation he is considering. Occasionally, the rigidity of these internal models may result in strong preconceptions which are extremely difficult to shake even in the light of conflicting evidence. At times, very weak organizational signals may be over-emphasized by a particular manager and far too much weight may be attached to their significance in subsequent decision-making. Conversely, organizational signals which would appear to demand immediate recognition and attention can sometimes be repeatedly overlooked in a manager's problem diagnosis.

Individual biases in change recognition

Biases and distortions of perception in recognizing and interpreting situations can occur for a wide range of reasons and these have been investigated for many years by psychologists in the rather artificial environment of the psychological laboratory. As yet, relatively little research has been conducted into the wider organizational aspects of this sort of perceptual distortion, although recently this practical problem has received increased attention. In his useful book *Judgement and Choice*, Robin Hogarth (1980) has catalogued many aspects of human judgemental fallibilities. Using an information-processing framework, this author has described many sources of bias in reasoning and linked these to the acquisition, processing, output and feedback stages of an individual's information processing strategies. Some of these are particularly relevant to the recognition of the need for organizational change and these are described below.

1. The availability of organizational signals This source of bias is concerned with the availability of particular sorts of evidence either from the manager's memory or from the immediate organizational environment. Often the importance of frequently discussed events is over-estimated since these loom large in a manager's memory and can be recalled more easily than equally important, though less well-publicized events. In a similar way managerial judgement can be affected by the perception of 'chance'

organizational cues and signals in the immediate organizational environment.
2. Selective perception This source of bias stems from several sources related
to the need to simplify the complexity of the real world. In an attempt to obtain
this order and consistency, managers structure events on the basis of their
own experience and consequently tend to seek information which is consistent with their own mental frameworks. This means that they often have a
tendency to see what they expect to see and to underplay conflicting evidence
which is not consistent with their own mental model.
3. The salience of concrete information This source of bias refers to the
frequently observed effect that concrete information dominates abstract information in managers' judgements. Managers tend to attach more weight to
information that has been based on their own or another's reported experience
than to information that is contained within reports or statistical summaries.
4. Illusory correlation or causality This source of bias stems from the
incorrect belief that two factors co-vary when in fact they do not or the incorrect belief that one factor causes another when this is not the case.
5. Conservatism in revising opinions This source of bias results from the
tendency of managers not to revise their opinions appropriately on the basis
of new information.
6. Use of 'heuristics' to reduce mental effort This source of bias is associated
with many attempts to apply 'rules of thumb' to organizational events and
situations. These strategies are popular since they reduce mental effort although
many sources of uncertainty are conveniently ignored. Such strategies include
stereotypic perceptions of organizational events, ignoring conflicting evidence
to achieve a supposed 'best guess', and basing conclusions on insufficient
evidence.
7. Environmental pressure This source of bias refers to the stress placed on
a manager by insufficient time, distractions, emotional stress and social or
political pressure. All of these factors can seriously impair the quality of a
manager's judgement.

Organizational conditions facilitating change recognition

However skilled the individual manager is in recognizing and defining the best
targets for change initiatives, there is little likelihood that he will be able to
be fully effective unless the structural and cultural features of the organization are conducive to his or her attempts to innovate. In addition to appropriate
individual conditions for effectively recognizing the need for change, there
is a range of organizational conditions which appear to be prerequisites for
active recognition of organizational problems and innovative decision-making.
Hopwood (1974) has outlined a number of these organizational conditions and
some of these are described below.

1. The problem-oriented organization needs to encourage the recognition of
problems and stimulate a diversity of ways in which to view them. This
development requires a richness and diversity of experience to foster the ability
to adapt to a changing environment.

2. The problem-oriented organization has decentralized authority and influence in order to encourage communication and debate across all levels and branches of the organization which are subsequently prompted to recognize and define potential organizational problems.

3. In the problem-oriented organization the role of the superior is more concerned with providing feedback and support and this superiority is authentic being based on superior expertise and knowledge.

4. In the problem-oriented organization managers are required to continually define and redefine their roles and responsibilities since structural 'looseness' is encouraged and departmentalization rejected as a promoter of parochialism.

5. In a problem-oriented organization there are fewer rules and procedures and rewards are not immediately dependent on formal status. These arrangements encourage initiative and enable alternative organizational practices to be freely considered.

It can be seen that the above listed organizational conditions are all essentially concerned with facilitating the discovery and recognition of organizational problems and ensuring the effective transfer of this information across traditional boundaries. It is illuminating to contrast these idealized innovation conditions with those organizational conditions currently being fostered by general managers in the NHS. The new managerialism has tended to reject any approach which smacks of the unfashionable human-relations perspective and has instead opted for a more heavily rational strategy where the emphasis is being placed on a tighter and more centralized control of objectives and their achievement together with the introduction of formal evaluation procedures. This hard-line stance has resulted as a direct response to the Government's desire to see health policies implemented without the diffusion of will and direction which had been identified by Griffiths as a major problem with the old consensus management arrangements. The ethos of tighter control is committed to attempts to emphasize individual accountability using detailed appraisals of deviations from anticipated levels of performance. Often these appraisals are narrowly financial and retrospective and tend to emphasize vertical rather than horizontal organizational relationships. The general manager's dilemma lies in balancing the desire to achieve organizational results using tighter organizational controls whilst recognizing the danger that these control strategies themselves are likely to stifle the dynamic flows of formal and informal information which is vital for ensuring the responsiveness of the organization to new change initiatives.

Searching for alternatives

We have seen that the neatly demarcated sequential stage approach to describing decision-making does not hold up too well in practice, although it does appear that a decision-maker's behaviour reflects the content, if not the strict sequence, of these stages. In reality, the manager's search for alternative courses of action does not necessarily follow or occur in isolation of the supposed earlier initial stages of problem recognition and definition. Managers often perceive problems and formulate potential solutions apparently simultaneously. In fact, the sequence of stages may be completely reversed with managers' championing preferred solutions prior to searching for and fitting these 'pet' schemes to organizational problems. In these cases, the availability and attraction of certain sorts of solution determines the problem recognition and definition activities.

The managerial search for alternative courses of action rarely proceeds in the systematic manner suggested by 'stage' theories of decision-making and, like the problem-recognition process, is characterized by a range of biases and constraints which serve the purpose of simplifying the process and reducing the effort expanded on this critical process. Typically, the search begins by looking for past precedents which can be perceived as similar to the current problem and past solutions may be seen as transferable and relevant to the new situation. The manager seeks familiar territory and the desire to reduce uncertainty may have the unfortunate effect of predisposing him/her to over-estimate the degree of similarity between the old and the new problem. If this appeal to precedent fails to generate many promising alternatives, the manager may expand his search to consider similar organizations and their apparently successful approaches to similar problems. The biases of wishful thinking may be in evidence here since managers may have a tendency to over-estimate the probability of desirable outcomes. If the search for similar cases is abandoned, managers will attempt to consider the actual presenting problem in terms of its links to the complex pattern of cause and effect relationships which characterize their own organization. Even at this point, these interrelationships may be simplified so that a rapid solution can be found.

Practically, it is often the case that the pressures on a general manager necessitate the curtailing of a full search for alternative courses of action and a specification of what the consequences of these alternatives might be. In these circumstances, particularly for the general manager who has an NHS background, the temptation is to fall back on supposed 'tried-and-tested' organizational practices. However, in a change-oriented organization it is vital that there is a real discontinuity with sub-optimal past procedures and practice and it is essential that general managers ensure that more active and creative searches for appropriate alternatives are undertaken.

Evaluating and selecting alternatives

The evaluation and selection of a final decision does not take place at the culmination of a logical process of decision-making. Rather, the evaluation of alternatives begins to take place as soon as they have been identified and an idea may either be dropped at this stage or pushed forward for further evaluation. The appraisal of any alternative involves both objective and subjective factors. Objective assessment involves the consideration of such issues as assessing the feasibility and cost-benefits of the option although these rational factors are by no means the only criteria by which a decision option is judged. Often subjective factors are equally if not more important in the decision as to whether any particular option is allowed to travel further along the road to possible selection. These subjective factors are linked to a manager's personal 'cost-benefit' analysis and draw upon his or her understanding of the political and cultural arena of which he or she is a part.

The ways in which general managers cope with the uncertainties of organizational life are only partly understood. Processes like decision-making and problem-solving do not have clear and unambiguous meanings in the real world of management. Making decisions and solving problems are the hallmark of much managerial work and probably rest upon the same mental mechanisms. Traditionally decision-making approaches have emphasized the selection and choice of alternative courses of action and problem-solving approaches have tended to stress information integration and mental syntheses in achieving a goal. Both aspects appear to be critical for the effective management of change.

General management as organizational problem-solving

Broadly defined, problem-solving in any context starts from a set of 'known' or 'givens', and involves the problem-solver making connections between this available evidence and 'unknowns' or 'conclusions'. Making these connections is a skilled mental activity which can be accomplished with varying degrees of creativity. Attempts to improve managers' problem-solving skills by training them in the application of creativity techniques to their organizational problems has become a substantial industry. Techniques such as brainstorming, force field analysis and lateral thinking have become well known to the management fraternity, and all of these are able to increase the sheer volume and apparent novelty of ideas brought to bear on organizational issues. Unfortunately, although many of these techniques are well-suited to increasing the frequency of novel ideas they do not provide any real means of evaluating the large number of diverse ideas generated in these sessions. As has been often observed they leave the manager with the problem of what to do with all of these novel approaches. It is clear that the key to effective problem-solving lies not merely in solution generation but also in the more complex area of solution evaluation. In making effective use of ideas a manager needs to draw upon his complex body of knowledge and experience which guides his understanding of a particular organizational situation and to relate this understanding to an appropriate strategy for change and from there to what he or she expects the future shape of the organization to be as a result of managerial interventions. This linking between what is perceived to be important in the current organizational 'problem-space' and finding effective solutions is only partly accomplished by generating possible solutions. In addition, the manager must evaluate these potential solutions by drawing on an understanding of the causes and consequences of organizational states and events.

The general manager who presents a rational case for change must justify (to himself and others) the connections he or she makes between current organizational 'evidence' and the conclusions which are drawn in erecting this conceptual linking network between current and future organizational states. This network of explanatory and predictive beliefs about organizational situations constitutes his or her working model of change. The problem-solving of general managers depends on the nature of the problem they have chosen for inclusion in their change agenda and the ways in which they prefer to select, conceptualize and tackle the issues which they have identified as key constructs in their view of the problem space. Although we would expect to observe different approaches to strategic decision-making and the wider process of managing change by different managers (and even by the same manager in different organizational situations), it seems reasonable to assume that similar stages in the change-management process should be evident across different managerial contexts. At some level the manager must be aware of the current organizational state and this awareness must have been gained informally or through more systematic efforts to diagnose the current organizational state. On the basis of this understanding, however imperfect or coloured by his own misconceptions or biases, the manager must design a strategy for implementing organizational change. The selected strategy will depend upon its anticipated utility in generating positive organizational outcomes. As the organizational state itself changes as a function of managerial intervention, the manager may evaluate these changes and choose to adapt his selected change strategy in order to 'tune' his strategy the better to meet his or her goals.

The working mental model of managers contains constructs which relate to these different phases of the change management process together with subjective theories about the relationship between these constructs. As we have previously argued, describing general managers' working models of change is of fundamental importance not only in understanding the change process itself but also in beginning to tackle the issue of managerial effectiveness. In order to understand managers' frames of reference towards organizational change, it is necessary to examine the managers' explanatory and predictive beliefs about organizational situations. From this perspective, managerial effectiveness is concerned with the content and compatibility of general managers' cognitive structures at each of the phases of change-management and is concerned with stressing the 'whys' of change as much as the traditional concerns with the 'whats' and 'hows' of change.

One theory of personality which has interesting implications for unifying organizational problem-solving, decision-making and creativity is the 'adaption-innovation' theory devised by Micheal Kirton (1987). Kirton has suggested that broadly there are two types of manager: those who are capable of initiating changes which improve the current system but who often fail to perceive new possibilities and, in contrast, those who are capable of generating ideas for radical change but who frequently fail in getting their ideas implemented. The first group is referred to as 'adaptors' and the second group is referred to as 'innovators'. Managers are suggested to lie somewhere along this bi-polar personality dimension which can be measured by examining the characteristic ways in which managers solve problems. The characteristic style which a manager uses in organizational problem-solving may be a useful summary device in aggregating the different underlying mental strategies which individual managers prefer to employ, although more research is necessary to further validate this hypothesized dimension.

Current approaches to mapping mental models

Recently there has been an upsurge of interest in the role of thinking in the individual manager's decision-making processes, particularly with respect to issue diagnosis and problem formulation. In a recent review Schwenk (1988) has discussed current research on strategic cognition and highlighted those topics which he considers to be most useful in understanding how decision-makers understand and solve strategic problems. In the past insufficient attention has been paid to the cognitive structures and processes of practising managers and much of the available evidence is grounded in academic cognitive psychology. However, Schwenk identifies two basic processes which appear to be at the heart of understanding the role of cognition in the strategic choice of managers. The first is the development of 'schemata' and the second is the application of these 'schemata' to the diagnosis of particular strategic problems. Schwenk has argued that there are two ways in which managers achieve understanding of strategic problems. For some problems, data may be carefully analyzed and an appropriate mental model developed. For others a previously developed mental model is transferred to the current organizational problem consequently saving effort and time in information search and diagnosis. As we have seen, distortions and biases appear to be prevalent in the development of managers' mental models and the application of old mental models to 'new' organizational problems may occur by the processes of 'analogy' and 'metaphor'. These processes by which a manager recognizes the opportunity for transferring an existing mental model to a new organizational domain have received some attention by researchers, but are not fully understood.

Part of the problem in theorizing about the development and application of mental models results from the lack of well-known methods to make these models explicit and available for examination and discussion. Some techniques are accessible and these include Axelrod's (1976) methods of cognitive mapping. These maps do not attempt to represent the individual's entire belief system, rather they represent the personal theories about a situation and attempt to make these explicit by providing a diagrammatic representation of the cause–effect relationships which the individual believes to exist between the variables of interest. Cognitive maps may be derived from a number of sources including decision documentation and interviews with decision-makers, and Bougon (1983) describes a method to elicit them. These methods are useful since they enable the underlying assumptions and consequences of any individual manager's perceptions to be explicitly examined.

Practically, what is required are techniques which enable the mental models of general managers to be represented in ways which demonstrate the relationships between organizational diagnosis, change strategy and expected outcomes. The cognitive mapping approaches are particularly valuable in highlighting the underlying assumptions and consequences of an individual's mental models but they are not specifically designed for investigating the management of change. However, there are a number of areas of research which are pertinent to the issues of change-management and which can provide useful inputs to its solution. The first area which can be usefully applied is managerial problem-solving.

Managerial problem-solving takes place within a 'problem-space' and this represents the manager's view of the problem to be solved and the actions necessary to search for a solution. The specific elements in the problem-space may or may not closely correspond to the elements in the organizational environment in which the solution strategy will be implemented. Problem-solving may take place with or without abstraction. When the task facing the manager is large and complex, the problem may be reformulated into more general and abstracted terms. Following the formation of an abstracted conceptualization or overview of the problem, the original problem may be partitioned into a series of smaller problems each of which may be solved in turn. Abstraction implies that the manager has developed an adequate understanding of the problem specifications so that the problem can be partitioned into sub-problems which can be tackled at the level of detail required to find a solution. In contrast problem-solving with no abstraction typically takes place with smaller, simpler problems, and in these instances the manager focuses on the generation, evaluation and execution of alternatives. Successful problem-solving for simpler problems requires effectively interacting with the environment in a more direct fashion.

The second dimension from the problem-solving area which is relevant to organizational interventions is what has been called the 'search-no-search' continuum. Search behaviour refers to the situation where there are a number of potential solutions and the manager's task is to select the most appropriate one from a set of alternatives. Typically search behaviour occurs where the manager has some understanding of the problem to be solved but does not have available a previously tried solution. In these instances the manager attempts to specify the types of possible solutions that will be considered by applying heuristics or 'rules-of-thumb' drawn from his knowledge and experience. In contrast, no-search behaviour occurs when the manager uses solutions that have been developed previously and which can be applied to the problem in hand because a similar problem has been encountered before.

Any manager's attempts to solve organizational problems can be guided by the nature of the problem itself or by his previous experience with similar problems. In other words the manager's behaviour may be data-driven or conceptually-driven and this is the third problem-solving dimension of interest. When a problem suggests the processes by which the solution is achieved, the manager typically becomes data-driven by focusing on detailed aspects of the organizational environment. In conceptually-driven behaviour the manager focuses efforts on attempting to understand the problem to be solved and selecting the goals and strategies which may prove appropriate and effective in the situation.

The second area of research which is particularly relevant to the mental model approach is personal construct theory. Kelly (1955) put forward the view that everyone is constantly engaged in categorizing similarities and differences which they perceive in their environment, and these categorizations are represented in an individual's mind as a set of bipolar categories. Since these categories refer to how an individual construes his environment these bipolar categorizations are usually called constructs. These constructs appear to be organized into complex networks in an individual's cognitive structures so that every individual possesses a unique set of organized constructs through which he or she perceives the world and by which he or she comes to make decisions about the most appropriate behaviour to use in dealing with current and future situations. Kelly has shown that these processes of categorization are a function of both individual and situational differences.

In other words in order to understand managers' frames of reference to organizational change it is initially necessary to discover the internal category structures they hold. These construct systems are the foundation for understanding how managers evaluate organizational states and identify methods of changing them. Techniques for eliciting construct systems, such as the widely-used Repertory Grid, may provide a means of assessing managerial effectiveness as change agents by allowing examination of construct appropriateness across a range of organizational situations.

The repertory grid technique has some particular advantages in that it focuses upon individual perceptions; it minimizes the potentially intrusive element of the researcher or investigator and can get below superficial descriptions of management tasks. As a flexible technique it can be applied to a range of situations and is thus a valuable tool in determining the content and structure of a manager's thoughts (Stewart and Stewart, 1976).

The third area of relevant research is case-study analysis. A case-study is usually concerned with examining an individual person in a particular situation. Practically, there are many different reasons for carrying out a case-study and the type of information required in the case-report can vary a great deal from one context to another. In fact, there is little general agreement on the content and organization of a case-study or on the specific procedures to be employed in examining individual people in situations. The development of a generally acceptable framework for the study of individual cases has been largely neglected and this has been partly due to limitations in the case-study approach. One of the main criticisms of the approach is that most case-studies are incomplete since one-sided accounts are included and equally acceptable alternative accounts are often not presented. Similarly, the explanatory concepts which are used to make sense of the individual's behaviour are often oversimplified and misleading. Frequently, people are summed up by using personality traits such as 'steady', 'dynamic', 'reliable' and so on. Clearly there is much more to a person than a few characteristic ways of behaving. Another deficiency stressed by critics of the case-study approach is that often the situational determinants of behaviour are not adequately emphasized, or the individual's own view of their circumstances, personal attributes and actions is not included. All of these criticisms are valid since the selection and interpretation of 'facts' about a person's motives and actions in a particular situation is never as straightforward as it might seem. Despite these criticisms of the case-study approach it remains a popular and useful means of capturing the richness and complexity of real-life managerial work. Although case material has often been 'thrown-in' to add human interest to dry accounts of managerial decision-making, if used properly it can provide real insight into complex managerial issues.

The real value of case-material is revealed when the structure of the case report is systematically analyzed. Case-reports tend to have a logical structure and to contain a range of different sorts of statement. These statements can refer to how an organizational problem arose, how the problem became known to management, what empirical facts were established, how these facts were interpreted, what conclusions were reached, what course of action was undertaken and so on. The logical structure of arguments in case-studies can be analyzed using a method developed by Toulmin (1958) who identified six basic components or types of statement in an argument and provided a means of structurally mapping these components. Analyzing case-studies in this way requires that the analyst makes inferences that go beyond the stated arguments since these are usually incomplete. The real benefit of Toulmin's approach is that it provides a means whereby the latent aspects of arguments can be made explicit.

Logical construct analysis

One way of approaching the problem of representing the mental models of managers is to examine case-studies of organizational change and to examine general managers' accounts of the focus, process and progress of their change strategies. Although case-studies can never be complete and are subject to biases of various kinds, valid insights can be gained if appropriate questions are asked of the case-study evidence and the answers subjected to analysis techniques which bring the structure of the managers' constructs about change into sharp focus. Logical Construct Analysis is a mapping technique which draws upon previous work into problem-solving, personal construct theory and case-study analysis and which we have devised to enable the structural representation of general managers' working models of change to be undertaken. The stages in the analysis are described and illustrated by their application to a case-study of general management which is included below.

Case-study: 'Creating   locality-based   health management'.

Male UGM	Age 42
Job title	Unit General Manager, Priority Services Unit
Previous job title	Unit Administrator – Acute, Maternal and Neonatal Services
Scope of unit	Priority Services Unit embraces the district services for mentally ill, mentally handicapped, elderly and all community services (1300 staff)

1. Focus of change

The DHA, in adopting the Griffiths philosophy, had supported the delegation of budgets and planning to reflect clinical priorities. With the support of his DGM and Chairman, the UGM felt he had a free hand in developing services along the lines of his and his colleagues' ideas. The UGM was aware of previous difficulties in the unit which stemmed from the partition of services into three overlapping divisions, which were not related to the Social Services boundary.

Consequently the focus of change was the creation of locally-based health management with the new divisions designed to coincide with the social services boundaries. In this restructuring, five locality managers were envisaged to run the service which was to be split into the following divisions.

(a) Services for the elderly
(b) Mental health services
(c) Mental handicap services
(d) Community services.

This approach was seen as potentially beneficial for the patient since it allows the development and provision of joint planning with local authorities enabling patient needs to be locally assessed and responded to. Joint-planning in this way was envisaged to facilitate the development of long-term working relationships between the health divisions and their counterparts in the social services, and this co-operation should make the transfer of funding and responsibilities easier. The UGM considered that the new general management ethos provided an ideal opportunity to deliver on issues which he suspected the system had previously inhibited.

2. The process of change

The change process was initiated by the UGM producing a document identifying proposals for the managment of the new unit and outlining the philosopy underlying the new provision. This document formed the basis for discussion at a number of staff meetings in order that ideas could be explored and comments and criticisms could be received. An open evening was organized to allow staff to participate in the debate and this was generally attended by members of the RCN.

Thirty-five written comments were received relating to the UGM's report and it became apparent that there was a great deal of tension and uncertainty amongst nursing staff about the proposals.

The UGM considered that his document discussing proposed changes was a useful 'sounding-board' for his ideal and enabled him to identify the political nature of many of the issues raised. Discussion with other UGMs in similar units was also seen as a useful way of clarifying these issues.

3. Evaluating progress to date

The UGM considered that his efforts to facilitate agreement to the new structure accelerated the achievement of change. This new structure is now mostly filled, the health-localities have been established and final moves of staff nearly accomplished.

The UGM feels that his approach has worked speedily and effectively. Despite the anxiety of the nurses, he considers his strategy of remaining 'detached' was correct since most of the nursing staff have been appointed to posts in the new structural arrangements.

The district has had a history of effective consultation and good working relations with medical staff and the UGM considered that this positive medical involvement would continue and was reflected by a GP member of the professional advisory group.

The objective of greater co-operation with the social services is now anticipated by the UGM rapidly to become a reality, enabling future priorities to be more effectively met.

Stages of logical construct analysis

Stage one: Statement identification

The first stage in the analysis is to identify the types of statement used in the case study arguments. Three types of statement have been found to be practically useful and these three are essentially Toulmin's data, claim and inference warrant categories, although for the sake of simplicity we prefer to call these categories, evidence, conclusion and justification statements respectively. These three types of statement form the 'units' of our analysis and are related as shown in figure 6.1.

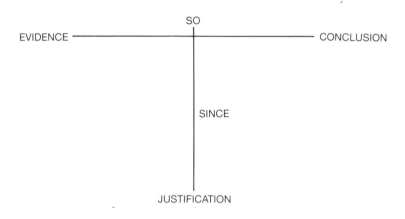

Figure 6.1   Units of analysis

Evidence statements are those which refer to what the general manager has used as the 'givens' or 'knowns' of his argument. Conclusion statements are those which the general manager sees as following from any statement of evidence. Consequently these two categories are related by the 'so' relationship as shown above. The third statement types is referred to as justification and identifies the general manager's reasons for the link between the evidence and the conclusion. Consequently the 'since' relationship characterizes the role of justification statements. Since arguments often proceed from the known to the unknown in a series of inferential stages, the conclusion from a piece of evidence can, in its turn, become a piece of evidence for a subsequent conclusion and so on. In other word, in accordance with Toulmin's approach, one and the same statement can function in different ways depending on how it is related to other statements in the case-study.

Table 6.1 shows the evidence, conclusion and justification statements contained in our case-study example and each identified statement is numbered. For ease of identification, identical statements which serve as both evidence and conclusion are coded with the same number.

It can be seen from the table that the trilogies of evidence, conclusion and

Table 6.1 Case-study – statement types

Evidence	Conclusions	Justifications
1. UGM had support of DGM and Chairman	2. UGM felt he had a free hand in developing services along his lines	
3. Services partitioned into overlapping divisions not related to social services boundaries	4. Difficulties in the unit	
4. Difficulties in the unit	5. Creation of locality-based health management (restructuring)	
5. Restructuring	6. Beneficial for patients	Joint planning enables patient needs to be locally assessed and reported to
5. Restructuring	7. Joint planning in new structure	
7. Joint planning in new structure	8. Facilities co-operative working relationships (co-operation)	
7. Joint planning in new structure	9. Transfer of resources easier	
8. Co-operation	9. Transfer of resources easier	
2. UGM felt he had a free hand in developing services along his lines	10. UGM produced change proposal document	Since new GM ethos provided the opportunity
10. UGM produced change proposal document	11. Opened arena for discussion	Change document useful sounding board for UGMs ideas
11. Opened arena for discussion	12. Nurses' tensions and anxieties revealed	
11. Opened arena for discussion	13. Political nature of many issues surfaced	
14. UGM efforts to facilitate agreement to new structure	15. Facilitates achievement of change	
16. UGM's 'detached' and objective approach	15. Facilitates achievement of change	

justification statements are sometimes incomplete. This is because managers often cite evidence which does not lead to a conclusion or evidence and conclusions are stated with no associated justification (reasonable or otherwise) for the inference. These missing components of the case for change are often as important as the reported statements in elucidating the structural deficiencies in general managers' working models of change. Of course, a number of components are implied rather than explicitly stated and these can be inferred from the case-study material. One of the primary purposes of Toulmin's approach to case-study analysis is to highlight the unstated assumptions of arguments in order to delve beneath the surface structure of case-studies. This depth of analysis can often prove useful although it raises the problem of the extent to which analysis can be validly pressed beyond the stated case-study arguments. For our purposes only the tabled statement types are used to provide a core understanding of the structure of general managers' working mental models of change.

Stage two: Relationship mapping

The table of statements begins to show the structure of the case study, but in order to make this structure more explicit each statement as well as being numbered is further coded into three categories representing the three broad phases of the process of organizational change. These are simply diagnosis of organizational state (category 'D'), strategy for change (category 'S'), or anticipated outcome (category 'O').

The next step is to arrange the identified statements into a circle as shown in Figure 6.2. Each pair of statements is considered from the point of view of whether the 'SO' relationship is used explicitly or implicitly to link them in the case-study of change. Arranging the statements in this 'anagram' fashion is an approach used by Glanville (1983) in his technique for uncovering the structure of students' learning concepts. Although our purpose is not the same as the 'anagram' approach, it is a useful visual aid in examining the relationships between different types of statements. It can be seen from the diagrammatic representation of the case-study above that the general manager's case for change can be traced through its causes and consequences as the manager sees it.

Stage three: Representing the model

The previous stage of the technique has provided a method of examining case study structure by using explicit and implicit coding of statement types and causal relationships (i.e. the 'SO' relationship). At this stage the three broad categories of the process of organizational change are used to provide the time dimension in our model. The diagram below arranges the statements into three types: diagnosis, strategy and outcome, and links them with the causal relationships identified in stage 2 of the technique. It is apparent from the model diagram that the 'SO' relationships, represented by directional arrows, can occur either within or between the three stages of the change process. The within stage relationships are useful in identifying separate 'concept clusters' within a manager's mental model of change whereas the between stage relationships enable the examination of the structure of the components which characterize each stage of the change process.

For the selected case-study example the diagram reveals two clusters of

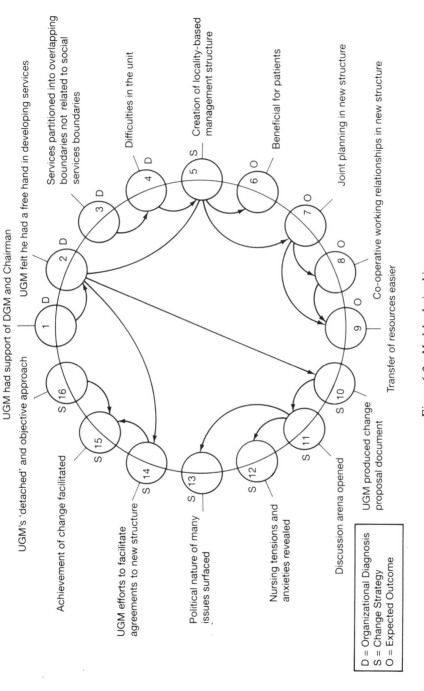

UGM had support of DGM and Chairman

UGM's 'detached' and objective approach

UGM felt he had a free hand in developing services

Services partitioned into overlapping boundaries not related to social services boundaries

Difficulties in the unit

Creation of locality-based management structure

Beneficial for patients

Joint planning in new structure

Co-operative working relationships in new structure

Transfer of resources easier

UGM produced change proposal document

Discussion arena opened

Nursing tensions and anxieties revealed

Political nature of many issues surfaced

UGM efforts to facilitate agreements to new structure

Achievement of change facilitated

1 D
2 D
3 D
4 D
5 S
6 O
7 O
8 O
9 O
10 S
11 S
12 S
13 S
14 S
15 S
16 S

D = Organizational Diagnosis
S = Change Strategy
O = Expected Outcome

Figure 6.2 Model relationships.

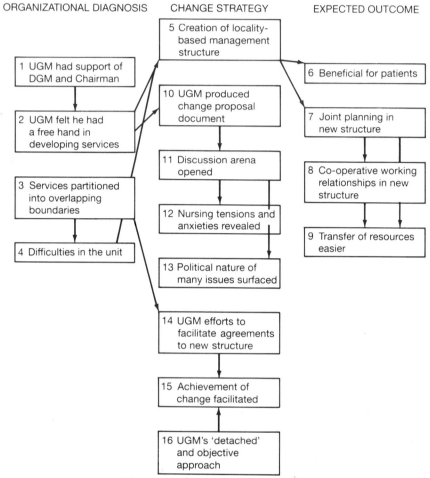

ORGANIZATIONAL DIAGNOSIS   CHANGE STRATEGY   EXPECTED OUTCOME

5 Creation of locality-based management structure

1 UGM had support of DGM and Chairman

6 Beneficial for patients

10 UGM produced change proposal document

2 UGM felt he had a free hand in developing services

7 Joint planning in new structure

11 Discussion arena opened

8 Co-operative working relationships in new structure

3 Services partitioned into overlapping boundaries

12 Nursing tensions and anxieties revealed

9 Transfer of resources easier

4 Difficulties in the unit

13 Political nature of many issues surfaced

14 UGM efforts to facilitate agreements to new structure

15 Achievement of change facilitated

16 UGM's 'detached' and objective approach

Figure 6.3 Change model representation

such concepts within the organizational diagnosis stage. The first cluster relates to the general manager's diagnosis of his own role which was characterized by the support and confidence of the DGM and chairman enabling him to feel he had a free hand in developing services. The second cluster relates to the general manager's diagnosis of the difficulties in the unit which he generally attributed to the fact that the services were partitioned into overlapping boundaries.

Within the second phase of the change process, change strategy, the diagram reveals three distinct clusters. Firstly, the core of the change strategy can be seen to be the creation of a locality-based management structure and this constitutes the first cluster. Secondly, the production of the change proposal document and its role in opening up discussion of many sensitive issues constitutes the second concept cluster. The third cluster is concerned with the objective and 'detached' approach which characterized the general manager's own efforts to facilitate agreement to the new organizational structure. For the third, expected outcome phase of the change process, there are two distinct clusters represented in the model. The first cluster is that the changes are expected to be beneficial for patients. The second cluster is more complex and is concerned with the benefits ensuing from the new arrangements which can be seen to be threefold: joint planning, co-operative working relationships and easier transfer of resources.

If we now turn our attention to the between stage relationships it is clear that the core of the change process as understood by the general manager is the creation of the new management structure which was facilitated by the recognition of the unit's difficulties and the general manager's own perception of support for his actions. This new structure is envisaged to have the twin benefits of being more effective for both patients and management. The other components of the change strategy are attempts to facilitate agreement to the new structure.

Stage four: Interpreting the model

The analysis of a general manager's approach to a particular organizational problem is not intended to provide a simplistic answer to the issue of effectiveness of change conceptualization or strategy; rather it is essentially a means of explicitly focusing upon an individual manager's mental model in a particular domain. There are a variety of specific ways in which the working models of change can be evaluated, but generally a model may be subject to two types of criticism. These can be called external criticism and internal criticism. External criticism arises from a comparison of the contents of the manager's model with the 'real' organizational features which the model is trying to represent. This type of criticism can only reliably come from other organizational members who have insight and understanding of the problem domain. On the other hand, internal criticism results from considering the logical structure of the model itself and is concerned with examining the logical consistency of the manager's conclusions and the explicit and implicit assumptions he has made in interpreting organizational evidence.

Some avenues for exploration are noted below and these are listed in the form of a number of questions. There are twenty-four questions organized under six categories. These are by no means exhaustive but attempt broadly to cover the important ground in approaching an evaluation of a general manager's approach to organizational change. These questions are concerned either with the structure or with the content of the manager's model. They are included here as a means of focusing attention on the interpretation of the outcome of the logical construct technique described above. The questions aim to highlight areas whereby the simplified models of the relationships relevant to the manager's perception of the change process can be further examined. In the next chapter a more structured change evaluation checklist is described and applied to several case-studies of change.

A useful starting point in questioning a manager's change strategy is often to look at the breadth and depth of the initial organizational diagnosis and to examine the evidence, assumptions and conclusions which the general manager has used to diagnose the organization as he sees it.

It is impossible for any general manager to focus upon all of the organizational information which may be pertinent to the organizational issue he or she wishes to consider. There is simply too much information and invariably not enough time to undertake an exhaustive data collection exercise. In practice, the manager has to be selective, and it is essential that he applies problem finding and problem defining skills in controlling his or her perception and understanding of the organization. We have seen earlier that scanning and focusing upon different aspects of the organization are dependent not only upon the current state of the organization but also upon how a general manager subjectively construes the meaning of the organization. Clearly, if an organization is confronting a crisis in one area it may appear to be inappropriate that the general manager is focusing his attention upon another, unless there are clear causal links between his anticipated point of intervention and the anticipated effects of the organizational change strategy. These links may not be always self-evident and it is essential that any attempt at evaluation is able to capture the anticipated flow of causes and consequences.

It is perfectly possible that a manager may have selected and adequately defined an appropriate organizational problem and has obtained appropriate and sufficient evidence to enable the nature of the problem to be evaluated. Unfortunately, it is all too common that reasonable conclusions have not been drawn from the evidence. Generally, there are two main causes for this type of failure in organizational diagnosis. Firstly, the manager may have preconceived notions about what the fundamental causes of the presenting problem are; in these instances the conclusions which may be drawn from the evidence are often biased. Secondly, the processes of actually making a reasonable judgement on what is always incomplete evidence may be difficult. In a complex situation, there is always the temptation to oversimplify reality in order that a reassuring impression of understanding and control can be engendered. Often this takes the form of a reluctance to consider evidence which may bring the manager's perception and understanding of an organizational issue into question. When a manager's mind is already made up, the likelihood of obtaining appropriate and sufficient evidence is severely curtailed. In these circumstances judgement is generally biased.

Evaluating approaches to organizational change

1. Adequacy of organizational diagnosis

(a) Has the manager selected and adequately defined an appropriate organizational problem?

(b) Has the manager obtained appropriate and sufficient evidence to evaluate the nature of the problem?

(c) Has the manager drawn reasonable conclusions from his evidence?

(d) Has the manager fully evaluated the ramifications of the relationships in his or her diagnosis?

2. Value of expected outcomes

(a) Are the expected outcomes realistically attainable?

(b) Are the expected outcomes worth pursuing?

    (c)   Do the expected outcomes have little or no appeal to any of the organizational interest groups?

    (d)   Has the manager considered the possibility of negative as well as positive outcomes?

3. Appropriateness of change strategy

    (a)   Has the manager considered the alternative change strategies?

    (b)   Does the selected change strategy seem appropriate?

    (c)   Is the selected change strategy practical?

    (d)   Does the process of implementation have little or no appeal to any of the organizational interest groups?

4. Compatibility of organizational diagnosis and change strategy

    (a)   Has the change strategy been specifically derived from the organizational diagnosis?

    (b)   Is the change strategy compatible with the organizational diagnosis?

    (c)   Are the justifications for the links between diagnosis and strategy reasonable or even apparent?

    (d)   Is the change strategy directly or indirectly linked to the organizational diagnosis?

5. Compatibility of change strategy and expected outcomes

    (a)   Are the expected outcomes specifically seen to result from the change strategy?

    (b)   Are the expected outcomes compatible with the change strategy adopted?

    (c)   Are the justifications for the links between strategy and expected outcomes reasonable or even apparent?

    (d)   Are the expected outcomes directly or indirectly linked to the change strategy adopted?

6. Explicit and implicit justifications

    (a)   Are the explicit justifications sensible?

    (b)   Does the model suggest underlying 'real' reasons rather than the 'good' reasons suggested?

    (c)   To what extent is the model a rationalization?

    (d)   Is the model distorted because of inappropriate justifications?

These types of questions enable a general manager's working model of change to be examined in greater detail. Often, it is necessary to question the adequacy of the case-study material, particularly if there are missing areas of interest. In these instances it is necessary to discover the information needed but this, of course, depends on the purposes for which the evaluation is to be put. The case-study used as an example here has been selected to illustrate the steps in using logical construct analysis with real material. Often the web of concepts, clusters, causes and consequences is more complex, but the technique's ability to analyze initial complexity into components makes it even more useful when a manager's motives are not immediately apparent.

CHAPTER 7
The pragmatics of change

We have seen that managers use mental models of their organizations to provide a framework through which they can view the process of change. The previous chapter has described some aspects of this subjective view of organizational reality and attempted to show how these perceptions affect and control managerial decision-making. The purpose of this chapter is to introduce a number of practical features of the organization which also need to be taken into account when considering organizational change. These features include the pressures and constraints on general managers, the importance of the ongoing organizational context and the central role of the individual manager's power and style in controlling and shaping the emerging organization. A change evaluation checklist is described which provides a means of systematically structuring the process of any particular organizational change, and this is related to several case-studies of change, included to illustrate some practical aspects of change management and its assessment.

Perceptions and performance

Many have argued that the public sector is fundamentally different from the business sector, not least because of the planning constraints inherent in pursuing statutorily defined activities. Business does not have these constraints and consequently is free to expand, contract and diversify its activities to maximize its profitability. Coupled with this requirement of meeting predefined objectives, the public sector has the associated problem of adequately measuring its goals and performance. The relatively simple business measures of profitability and rate of return on assets cannot be universally applied as the acid-test of performance in the public sector. Managers in the public sector must strike an appropriate balance between controlling costs and ensuring the 'quality' of service whilst simultaneously accommodating short-term political pressures which frequently run counter to good management practice.

However, the pressures on general managers in the NHS are not just political. Rosemary Stewart (1989) has recently listed what pressures and constraints DGMs perceive as acting upon them. Shortly after their appointment to these posts these pressures included uncertainties about the job demands and worries about their competence to do what was expected of them. Another source of uncertainty was lack of knowledge of the 'rules of the game', particularly with respect to their freedom to appoint and reorganize. These initial pressures have faded as job-familiarity has grown, but the on-going financial and political pressures remain and in some instances have recently increased. In addition to these pressures, a number of specific constraints on NHS general managers further differentiate them from the manager in the private sector. These perceived constraints include the inability of general managers to influence greatly the availability of money, to influence clinician's use of resources, the statutory requirements for a 'general' service and the nationally-determined pay and conditions for many of the staff. Specific characteristics such as these have prompted many to suggest that public sector management is quite different from business sector management.

However, this view of the uniqueness of public sector management is not by any means universally held. As Gunn (1989) has pointed out, many senior business executives would reject the notion that all their values, goals and quality of performance can be measured against the 'bottom line' of profitability and feel that they, like public sector managers, are equally the target of political pressure. In this case the political pressure emanates from business managers' accountability to investors, employees and customers. It may be that, despite the frequently debated differences between public and private sector management, there is a great deal more commonality than is often acknowledged. We have seen that there are many management processes and skills which are common to all managers, although the question of what managers actually do must be supplemented with an examination of a better understanding of why managers behave as they do.

Categories of change

It is abundantly clear that the pressures and constraints which general managers perceive are to a large extent subjectively defined since different managers may perceive an identical situation very differently depending upon their model of the managerial problem-space. These differing perceptions will affect the way in which managers select and define the organizational problems they target for action and this early formulization is crucial in determining the potential strategies for assessing the success or otherwise of their change strategies. If a specific and limited issue is defined, then measuring progress is made easier; conversely diffuse and generalized targets for change are less easily monitored, although these may prove to be equally if not more influential in engendering organizational success. The concept of service 'change' is vague and ill-defined and can refer to an extremely wide range of organizational innovations and transformations. However, there are several dimensions which can be used to categorize types of organizational change and a number of these have been previously discussed.

One simple, but useful, way of categorizing types of change has been used to examine the sorts of change which general managers were attempting to implement, and this has been described in Chapter 5. These categories are not mutually exclusive or even exhaustive but are at least relevant since they are those which our sample of general managers identified.

The different sorts of descriptors used in categorizing selected targets for change in the NHS has been debated by Pettigrew *et al.* (1989) who have argued that preoccupation with the intricacies of narrowly-defined changes is misleading since these can only represent static 'snapshots' of what is, in reality, a dynamic and holistic process. Pettigrew (1985) usefully distinguished the content or 'what' of change from both the process or 'how' of change and the context or 'why' of change. Context in this approach is very broadly defined and refers to national, economic and social factors as well as more localized aspects of strategy, structure, culture and so on. From this extremely broad and inclusive perspective the 'why' of change resides in a plethora of partially defined historical and social factors, although little attention is paid to the individual general manager as agent of change and even less to his or her values, motives and preferences. Pettigrew's expansive approach is broadly sociological and consequently pays scant regard to the perceptions and mental models of any individual agent of change. In our view, the individual manager and his or her mental structures and strategies are at the heart of an understanding of the interface between managers and professional groups. It is within the development of shared perceptions that the real indicators of the success of general management must lie. Overcoming the barriers between management and health care professionals requires that a shared view of what constitutes success is forged. Historical factors can help us understand many of the long-standing reasons for the mutual distrust between managers and clinicians but a better understanding of the psychological factors which maintain these conflicting perceptions is essential to the implementation and evaluation of organizational progress of change.

The individual manager and organizational control

A great deal has been written about the processes which govern and regulate organizational change and much of this has been in the realm of abstracted and academic theorizing. Often the change literature fails to capture the practical essence of change activities and scant attention has been paid to the practical role of the individual manager as the key agent of change within an organization. As we have seen, the real issues which Health Service managers must face are partly dependent on the nature of the organization itself and partly dependent upon the model of the organization which the manager uses to define and interact with these organizational issues. Human behaviour is largely unpredictable and does not conform to the regularities of many proposed systems, and this lack of predictability is exacerbated by too narrow an emphasis of many approaches. Although much has been made of the micro-politics of organizational change, relatively little attention has been focussed on the personal and individual cognitive structures of managers themselves.

The effectiveness of a general manager in shaping change depends upon the adequacy of the mental models which he/she is employing and upon the ability to act upon these models in implementing his change agenda. In other words a manager must possess the skills to build or adapt his mental models through the learning process and to translate what he has learned to guide his/her organizational behaviour. Human and social factors are clearly of great importance in this process and the effective manager needs to make some working assumptions about the ways in which people are motivated, and how these assumptions relate to the realities of power, influence and control in the organization.

The complexity and uncertainty which characterizes life in a large enterprise like the NHS can appear to present insurmountable difficulties to anyone who is attempting to understand the dynamics of the organization. It is clear that, despite the inevitable conflicts and power-struggles which occur, the processes by which the overall direction and control of the organization is maintained are purposeful and well co-ordinated. These processes are not easy to describe and many specialist approaches have superimposed their own models and terms of reference onto the many-faceted problems of organizational dynamics. Sociologists and psychologists have tackled the problem of control from the social and interpersonal perspective, whereas those with a more mechanistic bent have attempted to represent whole enterprises as controlled cybernetic systems.

Unfortunately, the numerous efforts in this area have not resulted in any complete description of the processes of organizational control. Increasingly, it is being realized that there is an important distinction between the design and development of specific organizational controls (e.g. performance review schemes, information reporting systems, job descriptions, budgetary reviews and so on) and the general aim of ensuring purposeful control of the organization as a whole. This apparent paradox results from a range of factors, not least the problem which Merton described in his pioneering work published in 1957. Merton emphasized that senior managers' desire to control organizations has its origins in subjective and personal factors and although these are rapidly translated into organizational terms, they frequently result in the introduction of specific control schemes. One of the main purposes of these control schemes is to ensure that the consequences of subordinate managers' behaviour becomes more visible, enabling senior management to operate the 'management by exception' strategy. Consequently, the managerial emphasis has then shifted to evaluating subordinate managers on the basis of the organizational rules based on these control schemes rather than evaluating the efforts and the effectiveness of the individual managers concerned. As the variety of specific control schemes proliferates it is in the subordinate managers' interests to find the easiest rather than the most effective means of satisfying them. 'Playing the organizational game' becomes an end in itself and as a consequence managerial behaviour becomes increasingly rigid and defensive. The organization's ability to respond to change declines and senior managers may embark on the downward spiral of introducing further controls in an attempt to rectify the situation.

This sort of scenario may have a parallel in recent performance appraisal initiatives undertaken in the NHS. The Individual Performance Review (IPR) appraisal scheme which has been introduced at the higher and middle managerial tiers of the NHS has been welcomed by many, although others have expressed the concern that reducing managerial work to a list of tasks may have the unanticipated effect of these tasks being followed too closely, resulting in managers rigidly pursuing these tasks at the expense of the real objectives of effectiveness. In a complex environment like the NHS it is much easier to set minimum rather than effective standards of performance since the latter requires managerial flexibility and adaptation to the organizational environment which cannot be easily quantified or anticipated.

Power and role

The extent to which specific systems of organizational control are introduced by management is not simply determined by the desire of senior managers to improve predictability but are also frequently seen as a means of extending and legitimizing the power which senior management wields. Formalizing the managerial control mechanisms into specific schemes may reduce the extent to which senior managers need to use overt power for control purposes, but the introduction of such impersonal devices may also have the unanticipated effects of increasing the perceived level of threat and alienating subordinate staff. General managers must understand how to use power as a means of influencing organizational change if they are to be effective. The misplaced desire simply to increase the predictability of their subordinates' behaviour may stem from a wide range of factors. One of these may be their own perceived powerlessness in influencing the organization. We have seen that general managers in the NHS perceive that they are restricted by a range of constraints that their counterparts in business are not subjected to. These constraints include limited freedom to control the use of medical expenditure, limited ability directly to influence available capital or revenue, and restricted scope for influencing pay and conditions for staff. These constraints are real and may result in a perception of powerlessness in these problematic areas. However, this felt powerlessness may spread to the wider spectrum of a general manager's activities, ultimately eroding their belief that significant organizational change is a practical possibility.

Fortunately, there are sources of power which the general manager can draw upon and two of these appear to be particularly pertinent to the current situation. These are the areas of connection power and role power. Connection power is the power which a general manager holds as a function of social access and network membership throughout all levels of the organization. If a general manager's role is well connected to other roles in the organization, then effectiveness will be increased since there is likely to be a joint effort to understand organizational problems and co-operative attempts to seek appropriate solutions. We have seen that building and maintaining networks of contacts both within and outside the organization is one of the hallmarks of managerial work and one of the main ways in which acceptance and facilitation of change is made possible.

The concept of 'role' has been variously described but has often been used to provide a 'handle' on the consideration of managerial effectiveness. General managers require job knowledge and skills to perform effectively but on its own this level of competence is not sufficient to ensure managerial effectiveness. In addition it is necessary that their role allows this competence to be expressed. Plant (1987) has argued that most managers do not adequately fill their roles since they are unwilling to exercise the power that their role legitimately allows them to display. This constraint on the exercise of legitimate power is often self-imposed and can occur for a variety of reasons. One important factor relates to the degree of confidence that a manager feels in the areas he is operating in and we have seen that this lack of confidence is prevalent when a general manager has been recently appointed. The Templeton tracer studies followed the progress of twenty DGMs in England and Wales from the spring of 1985 and found that this sample of managers was subject to numerous uncertainties about the scope of their roles and consequently were not confident in pursuing a number of legitimate goals. Another factor in delimiting the potential role effectiveness of general managers is the personal bias which managers choose to use when attempting to influence others. These managerial styles reveal a great deal about the model of the organization with which a manager views his or her organization and are considered in a little more detail in the next section.

Preferred managerial styles

It has been frequently observed that two managers may tackle similar organizational problems with ostensibly the same strategy and yet achieve radically different results. What appears to differentiate successful from unsuccessful managerial interventions is the approach or style that the particular manager chooses to use. It has been repeatedly emphasized by many influential management commentators that the task of management can never be accomplished by simply considering the technical aspects of managerial tasks in isolation. The effective control of any enterprise requires that the pressures exerted by individuals over one another also need to be taken into account. These informal mechanisms of social control are crucial since there is always a social relationship between managers and their subordinates and the personalities, preferred work styles and degree of acceptance of managerial authority all play an influential part in determining the outcomes of managerial interventions.

Many writers have produced extensive recommendations on how to manage the human side of the enterprise and the well-known approach of Blake and Mouton, for example, classifies management style on the basis of two dimensions, concern for people and concern for the task. Not surprisingly, the combination of a high concern for both is seen as maximizing both human and economic results. Likert has produced a similar four-fold classification of management style and suggests that a participative and group-oriented style of management is preferable.

The individual manager is of fundamental importance in shaping the course of events to bring about change within his or her organization. Much has been written about what distinguishes an effective from an ineffective manager and this has been typically tackled from the contrasting viewpoints of managerial behaviour (i.e. what managers do) and managers' managerial characteristics (i.e. what traits managers possess). We have seen in an earlier chapter that effective general managers tend to be emotionally stable achievers with good interpersonal and communication skills. In a changeable environment, they must also be open and adaptable to new ideas and approaches.

In the turbulent climate of the NHS, day-to-day work pressures often necessitate that managers take rapid action without the benefit of sufficient time and effort being spent in diagnosing the current organizational state and planning for change. Often, this pressure to perform suits many managers' action-oriented style since these types of managers would prefer to invest their effort into 'getting on with the job', rather than spend time on analyzing and reflecting upon the nature of the organizational problem and identify the potential strategies which may be available to reach a solution. Conversely, a manager who spends too long in contemplation may do so at the expense of timely and effective action. An effective manager is one who not only possesses appropriate job knowledge and skills but also has structured his or her role to enable their particular areas of competence to be effectively applied in the organizational context. In this sense, a manager's role is the mechanism by which knowledge and skills are transferred to managerial behaviour. To maximize effectiveness, the manager's role should provide sufficient opportunities for using those transferable experiences, specialized knowledge and managerial skills which are the individual manager's forte. An effective general manager is more likely to have carved out a role which enables him to demonstrate his or her particular talents than an equally competent manager who has not structured his or her role appropriately.

Of course, an effective role cannot simply be a vehicle for idiosyncratic aptitudes but must also take account of wider goals and objectives beyond the individual manager's purely parochial concerns. The effective general manager's role should also enable broader organizational goals to be met and this invariably entails co-operation and collaboration with many others in confronting organizational issues. In order to meet organizational objectives, the general manager must exercise his or her influence over others. Plant (1987) describes four types of influencing styles and suggests that the effective manager utilizes a broad spread of styles by matching styles to situation. These four styles are assertive persuasion, reward and punishment, common vision and participation and trust. We have organized the four styles which Plant outlines into a four-fold classification as shown below.

	EMOTIONAL	RATIONAL
COMPETITIVE	Contingency style	Reasoning style
CO-OPERATIVE	Visionary style	Participatory style

The contingency style of management is characterized by the use of rewards and punishments, whereby the manager presents clear and specific statements of what is required from subordinates. This is a competitive style since the underlying philosophy is to 'push' subordinates to better performance levels using the power and authority of the manager's position. The contingency style is an emotional one since it depends upon the twin tools of praise and criticism and these are directed toward the individuals performing the task.

In contrast to the contingency style of management, the reasoning style attempts to appeal to the rational rather than the emotional side of those who are being influenced. Like the contingency style, it is a competitive approach but ideas and arguments rather than individuals are rewarded and punished.

The manager who uses this style enjoys active discussion and debate and marshalls logic, facts and opinions to assert his viewpoint.

Unlike the competitive and reasoning styles of influence, the visionary style is based upon co-operation and entails the manager in the process of mobilizing energy and resources by appealing to the hopes, values and aspirations of others. Like the contingency approach, the visionary style of influence is aimed at appealing to others' emotions but it does so by drawing others into a shared vision of the exciting possibilities to come.

The participatory style is based on rational co-operation and is characterized by mutual trust and openness to others. The contributions of others to achieving organizational goals is freely discussed and the resources relevant to task achievement are rationally allocated.

These categories of influencing style have some face validity but which style or combination of styles is most appropriate in particular management situations is more difficult to disentangle and requires a greater understanding of the underlying dimensions which underpin management situations. As we have seen, one potentially useful way in which to begin to make some inroads into classifying management situations is to examine the process of organizational change from the perspective of how the organization is understood by managers. In the next section we describe a change evaluation checklist which attempts to provide a structured way of examining the management of organizational change from a process perspective.

Evaluating the management of change

We have seen that change management can be usefully, if somewhat over-simplistically, conceived as a three-stage process. These three stages are: diagnosis of organizational problem, adoption of change strategy and evaluation of outcomes of change. At the early stages of a programme of change, the actual outcomes of the change process are not yet apparent and initially these outcomes are merely expected or anticipated. As the change strategy is implemented, the actual change outcomes begin to become apparent and these can then be classified as either intended or unintended outcomes.

In attempting to understand a particular case-study of change, it is essential to consider two distinct aspects of evaluation. These aspects are firstly, the type of approach which management adopts at each of the three stages and secondly, the adequacy of the approach at each of the same three stages. Type of approach is concerned with identifying what sorts of issues and strategies have been selected and to what extent these have influenced the organization. Adequacy of approach is concerned with the effectiveness of these approaches and their validity and compatibility within the management of change.

It can be seen from table 7.1 that type of approach can be seen to consist of two main areas, which are labelled focus and impact. Focus is concerned with the range of social, political, cultural and structural factors which management may or may not take into account at each of the three stages of the change process. Impact is concerned with the different aspects of management's adopted approach which may influence the organization to a greater or lesser

Table 7.1 Twelve areas of evaluation

Change process	TYPE (Focus and impact)	ADEQUACY (Effectiveness and compatibility)
Problem diagnosis	What sorts of approaches are being or have been adopted in the diagnosis of the organizational problem?	How well executed are or will be the processes of organizational diagnosis?
	What is the impact of these problem-diagnostic activities upon the organizational sub-systems?	How compatible is the problem diagnosis with the scale and type of organizational problem?
Change strategy	What sorts of approaches are being or have been adopted to implement organizational change?	How valid and effective is the proposed or actual change strategy?
	What is the impact of the change strategy upon the organizational sub-systems?	How compatible is the change strategy with the level and type of problem diagnosis?
Outcomes of change	What sorts of change outcome are expected to occur or have resulted from the change programme?	How valid and useful are the expected or actual outcomes of the change programme?
	What is the impact of the outcomes of change upon the organizational sub-systems?	How compatible are the outcomes of change with the problem diagnosis and change strategy?

extent. This influence may be reflected in such factors as use of resources, involvement of staff and the vigour with which management pursues its change agenda. Similarly, adequacy of approach can be seen to consist of two broad areas, which are labelled effectiveness and compatibility. Effectiveness is concerned with how well the selected management approaches are executed and compatibility is concerned with the appropriateness of the management approach and the extent to which each of the stages of the change process are 'matched' with other stages. The table illustrates the twelve areas where evaluation of a change programme should be considered.

Each of the twelve areas of evaluation can be tackled at a variety of levels of detail and complexity. One simple approach is to use a checklist of features which can be applied to any case-study of change. One such checklist is included here and the advantage of this broad descriptive form of evaluation is that it enables the characteristic features of any change attempt to be explicitly described in a way which enables it to be compared with other case-studies of change.

The change evaluation checklist

How to complete the checklist

The purpose of this checklist is to give you the opportunity of evaluating a planned, on-going or recently completed programme of organizational change.

In the spaces provided at the top of the checklist please write your name, your job-title, the date and a brief identifying description of the change programme you intend to evaluate.

The checklist consists of fourteen statements in each of six evaluation areas resulting in 84 statements in all. In the light of what you know about the change programme, you are asked to state whether you agree or disagree with each of the statements. You must always choose either 'A' or 'D' for each statement even if this means that you have to make inferences or go beyond the evidence you have about the change programme in question.

If you agree with a statement then circle the letter 'A' next to the statement. If you disagree with a statement then circle the letter 'D' next to the statement. However, if you feel that you do not have enough evidence to confidently justify your choice, then in addition to circling 'A' or 'D', circle the letter 'U' for that particular statement. 'U' stands for uncertain.

Work at your own pace and remember there are no right or wrong answers. Try to ensure that you rate all of the 84 statements as either 'A' or 'D' and do so in the way which best represents what you feel about the change programme you are evaluating.

NAME: DATE:
JOB-TITLE:
BRIEF DESCRIPTION OF CHANGE PROGRAMME:

(TP) Type of problem diagnosis

For this programme of change, do you agree or disagree with the following statements about the type of problem diagnosis which has or will be undertaken by management

1. TP–I: The problem diagnosis is essentially a reaction to a perceived opportunity or threat	A D U
2. TP–R: The problem diagnosis takes account of assessing political factors (i.e. preferences, goals and strategies of interest groups and dominant coalitions)	A D U
3. TP–R: The problem diagnosis takes account of assessing the formal organizational arrangements (i.e. structure and operating systems)	A D U
4. TP–I: The problem diagnosis uses a substantial amount of organizational resources	A D U
5. TP–R: The problem diagnosis takes account of assessing the organizational culture (i.e. shared values and norms)	A D U
6. TP–I: The problem diagnosis is mainly focused on a well-focused organizational issue rather than on a diffuse organizational 'syndrome'	A D U
7. TP–I: The problem diagnosis is essentially proactive and in anticipation of new events or situations	A D U
8. TP–R: The problem diagnosis takes account of assessing the external environmental factors (e.g. demographics, political pressure and public attitudes)	A D U

9.	TP–I:	The problem diagnosis takes account of a large amount of organizational data and information	A	D	U
10.	TP–R:	The problem diagnosis takes account of assessing human assets (i.e. skills, abilities, expectations)	A	D	U
11.	TP–R:	The problem diagnosis takes account of assessing tangible assets (i.e. land, buildings equipment)	A	D	U
12.	TP–I:	The problem diagnosis involves many personnel in assessing organizational information	A	D	U
13.	TP–R:	The problem diagnosis takes account of assessing the social structure of the organization (i.e. relationships of power and affiliation)	A	D	U
14.	TP–I:	The problem diagnosis involves a great deal of communication with many members of the organization	A	D	U

(AP) Adequacy of problem diagnosis

For this programme of change, do you agree or disagree with the following statements about the adequacy of the process of problem diagnosis which has or will be undertaken by management

15.	AP–E:	Broadly, the problem diagnosis is characterized by effective communication with all the interest groups and dominant coalitions	A	D	U
16.	AP–C:	Essentially the selected organizational problem is well defined and understood by the diagnostic process	A	D	U
17.	AP–E:	Broadly, the problem diagnosis is not characterized by an over-simplification of some of the more important issues	A	D	U
18.	AP–C:	The problem diagnosis has adequately considered all the important ramifications of the problem	A	D	U
19.	AP–E:	Broadly, the problem diagnosis is not characterized by an over-elaboration of some of the less important issues	A	D	U
20.	AP–E:	Broadly, the problem diagnosis is not characterized by over- or under-weighting of the importance of some key organizational variables	A	D	U
21.	AP–C:	Broadly, the problem diagnosis is characterized by encouraging and co-ordinating others to search for, recognize and define problem areas	A	D	U
22.	AP–E:	Broadly, the problem diagnosis is characterized by the effective analysis of internal organizational evidence	A	D	U
23.	AP–C:	Essentially an appropriate organizational problem is selected for diagnosis	A	D	U
24.	AP–E:	Broadly, the problem diagnosis is characterized by the effective analysis of external environmental evidence	A	D	U
25.	AP–C:	The amount of resources used in problem diagnosis is broadly in step with the importance of the problem	A	D	U
26.	AP–E:	Broadly, the problem diagnosis is characterized by an active and extensive search for potential problem areas	A	D	U

27. AP–C: Those personnel directly involved in making the problem diagnosis are the most suitable for this activity A   D   U
28. AP–C: The problem diagnosis considers an appropriate
balance and 'mix' of organizational issues   A   D   U

(TC) Type of change strategy

For this programme of change, do you agree or disagree with the following statements
about the type of change strategy which has or will be adopted by management

29. TC–R: The change strategy is directed at changing
formal organizational arrangements (i.e. structure
and operating systems)   A   D   U
30. TC–I: The change strategy is essential aimed at fast organizational change rather than slow organizational change   A   D   U
31. TC–I: The change strategy is essentially aimed at large-
scale organizational change rather than small-scale
organizational change   A   D   U
32. TC–R: The change strategy is directed at changing
human assets (i.e. skills, abilities, expectations)   A   D   U
33. TC–I: The change strategy is more of an incremental ('step-
by-step') strategy than a radical ('big-leap') strategy A   D   U
34. TC–R: The change strategy is directed at changing the
social structure of the organization (i.e. relationships of power and affiliation)   A   D   U
35. TC–I: The change strategy is directed at changing
tangible assets (i.e. land, buildings, equipment)   A   D   U
36. TC–I: The change strategy takes a great deal of time to
implement   A   D   U
37. TC–R: The change strategy is directed at changing the
organizational culture (i.e. shared values and norms)   A   D   U
38. TC–I: The change strategy requires a large amount of
resources to implement   A   D   U
39. TC–R: The change strategy is directed at changing
political factors (i.e. goals and strategies of
interest groups and dominant coalitions)   A   D   U
40. TC–I: Implementing the change strategy requires a large
number of personnel to become actively involved   A   D   U
41. TC–I: Implementing the change strategy has a
widespread effect upon the organization   A   D   U
42. TC–R: The change strategy is directed at changing
external environmental factors (e.g. expectations,
political pressure and public attitudes)   A   D   U

(AC) Adequacy of change strategy

For this programme of change, do you agree or disagree with the following
statements about the adequacy of the change strategy which has or will be adopted
by management

43. AC–E: The change strategy takes adequate account of
the social dimensions of implementing change   A   D   U
44. AC–C: The change strategy is selected from an
appropriate range of considered alternatives   A   D   U
45. AC–E: The change strategy takes adequate account of

	the political dimensions of implementing change	A	D	U
46. AC–C:	The amount of resources used in implementing the change strategy are broadly in step with the scale of the change programme	A	D	U
47. AC–E:	The implementation of the change strategy is adequately planned	A	D	U
48. AC–C:	Generally, the change strategy is acceptable to all the main interest groups or coalitions	A	D	U
49. AC–C:	Broadly, the change strategy is clearly derived from, and compatible with the problem diagnosis	A	D	U
50. AC–E:	Broadly, the change strategy is characterized by an active and adaptive approach to its implementation	A	D	U
51. AC–C:	Those directly involved with implementing change are the most appropriate for this change programme	A	D	U
52. AC–E:	Essentially the change strategy is realistic and practical to implement	A	D	U
53. AC–E:	Broadly, the implementation of the change strategy engenders confidence and commitment	A	D	U
54. AC–C:	Implementing the change strategy does not engender unrealistic expectations of organizational interest groups	A	D	U
55. AC–E:	The change strategy takes adequate account of the behavioural dimensions of implementing change	A	D	U
56. AC–C:	Implementing the change strategy does not engender excessive demands on the organizational capabilities	A	D	U

(TO) Types of outcomes of change

For this programme of change, do you agree or disagree with the following statements about the types of outcomes of change which are or will be a consequence of the change strategy adopted by management

57. TO–I:	The early outcomes of change are catalysts for further intended change	A	D	U
58. TO–R:	The outcomes of change are mainly apparent in organizational arrangements (i.e. structure and operating systems)	A	D	U
59. TO–I:	The outcomes of change have a significant effect on the organization	A	D	U
60. TO–R:	The outcomes of change are mainly apparent in political factors (i.e. preferences, goals and strategies of interest groups and dominant coalitions)	A	D	U
61. TO–R:	The outcomes of change are mainly apparent in human assets (i.e. skills, abilities, expectations)	A	D	U
62. TO–I:	The early outcomes of change are catalysts for further unintended change	A	D	U
63. TO–I:	The outcomes of change have a significant effect on a large number of personnel	A	D	U

64.	TO–R:	The outcomes of change are mainly apparent in external environmental factors (e.g. demographics, political pressure and public attitudes)	A	D	U
65.	TO–R:	The outcomes of change are mainly apparent in tangible assets (i.e. land, buildings, equipment)	A	D	U
66.	TO–I:	On the whole, the outcomes of change are more intentional than unintentional	A	D	U
67.	TO–R:	The outcomes of change are mainly apparent in the social structure of the organization (i.e. relationships of power and affiliation)	A	D	U
68.	TO–I:	Assessing the outcomes of change requires taking account of a large amount of organizational information	A	D	U
69.	TO–R:	The outcomes of change are mainly apparent in the organizational culture (i.e. shared values and norms)	A	D	U
70.	TO–I:	Assessing the outcomes of change requires a significant number of personnel in collecting, collating and analyzing organizational information	A	D	U

(AO) Adequacy of outcomes of change

For this programme of change, do you agree or disagree with the following statements about the adequacy of the expected outcomes of change which are or will be a consequence of the change strategy adopted by management

71.	AO–E:	The outcomes of change have not created further sources of ineffectiveness	A	D	U
72.	AO–C:	The outcomes of change are valued by all interest groups or coalitions	A	D	U
73.	AO–E:	The outcomes of change justify the change strategy adopted	A	D	U
74.	AO–E:	The outcomes of change are clearly beneficial to the organization	A	D	U
75.	AO–C:	The outcomes of change are clearly linked to and broadly compatible with the original problem diagnosis	A	D	U
76.	AO–E:	On the whole, the outcomes of change are realistically attainable	A	D	U
77.	AO–C:	The assessment of the outcomes of change has used appropriate organizational information	A	D	U
78.	AO–E:	The outcomes of change have successfully eliminated some sources of ineffectiveness	A	D	U
79.	AO–E:	The outcomes of change are validly measured and monitored	A	D	U
80.	AO–E:	On the whole, the anticipated outcomes of change are worth pursuing	A	D	U
81.	AO–C:	Those directly involved in assessing the outcomes of change are the most suitable for this activity	A	D	U
82.	AO–C:	The outcomes of change are clearly linked to and broadly compatible with the change strategy	A	D	U

83.	AO–C:	The amount of resources used in assessing the outcomes of change are broadly in step with the scale of the change strategy	A	D	U
84.	AO–C:	The outcomes of change are used to adapt or 'tune' the on-going change strategy	A	D	U

Scoring the checklist

The checklist consists of six sections with fourteen statements within each section.

TP:	Type of problem diagnosis:	Statements 1–14
AP:	Adequacy of problem diagnosis:	Statements 15–28
TC:	Type of change strategy:	Statements 29–42
AC:	Adequacy of change strategy:	Statements 43–56
TO:	Type of outcomes of change:	Statements 57–70
AO:	Adequacy of outcomes of change:	Statements 71–84

Each of the six sections contains two sorts of statement. Within the three 'type' sections (i.e. TP, TC and TO) half of the statements in each section are 'range' (R) statements and the other half of the statements are 'impact' (I) statements. There are therefore seven 'range' statements and seven 'impact' statements in each of the three 'type' sections.

Similarly, within the three 'adequacy' sections (i.e. AP, AC and AO) half of the statements are 'effectiveness' (E) statements and the other half are 'compatibility' (C) statements. There are therefore seven 'effectiveness' statements and seven 'compatibility' statements in each of the three 'adequacy' sections.

In addition to being numbered, each of the statements in the checklist is coded. For example, the following two statements are coded AP–E and TC–I respectively. Consequently statement 20 is an adequacy of problem diagnosis/effectiveness statement and state 41 is a type of change strategy/impact statement.

20.	AP–E:	Broadly, the problem diagnosis is not characterized by over- and under-weighting of the importance of some key organizational variables	A	D	U
41.	TC–I:	Implementing the change strategy has a widespread influence upon the organization	A	D	U

In order to score your completed checklist simply add up all the times you have agreed with a statement (i.e. circled 'A') in each of the twelve categories. Each of these twelve categories can have a value of between 0 and 7 and is entered into a table like the one shown below. In addition to all the statements being rated as either agree or disagree, the evaluator has the option of signifying if he or she is uncertain of any of the choices by additionally circling the 'U' next to any statement. This level of uncertainty is also determined by adding up all the times 'U' has been circled in each of the twelve categories. Each of these twelve uncertainty scores can have a value between 0 and 7 and these are also entered into the table.

Table 7.2 shows an example of the scores which may be obtained by applying the checklist to a particular programme of organizational change.

Table 7.2   Example profile of management of change programme

	Problem diagnosis		Change strategy		Outcomes of change	
(0–7)	PD	U	CS	U	OC	U
Range –R	7	1	3	1	2	3
Impact –I	2	2	1	2	1	4
Effectiveness –E	6	1	1	0	1	6
Compatibility –C	3	2	1	1	1	5

The pattern of the scores within and between categories can be considered a 'profile' of the management of the change programme under consideration. In the example shown in the table above, we can see that this hypothetical change programme is characterized by a very wide-ranging problem diagnosis (score of 7) which has not had a great deal of impact upon the organizational sub-systems (score of 2). These problem diagnostic activities were well executed (score of 6) but were not seen by the evaluator as being particularly compatible with the scale and type of organizational problem (score of 3). Turning to the second strategy phase of the process, we can see from the table that although there was a moderate range of approaches inherent in the change strategy are both seen as low (scores of 1 for both). The last but one column of the table shows us that the outcomes of change are restricted in their range, impact, effectiveness and compatibility (respective scores of 2, 1, 1 and 1). An examination of the spread of the uncertainty scores on the table suggests that the evaluator is fairly confident in his assessment of both the problem diagnosis and change strategy phases but is less confident with respect to his assessment of the outcomes of change. This uncertainty may be due to the unavailability of evidence about the outcomes of change.

The checklist has been applied to each of the five case studies which are described below, and a graphical summary has been included for each one. Since this sort of broad evaluation partly depends on the evaluator's interpretation of organizational events, you may like to compare your evaluation with ours, in order to highlight areas of agreement and disagreement.

For the sake of brevity, shortened forms of the five case studies are included followed by a graphical summary based upon our application of the checklist to each case study in turn.

For the sake of simplicity, a mean uncertainty score was calculated for each of the three stages of the change process and these are shown on each of the graphs.

The case studies of change

A small sub-sample of managers were interviewed in depth to provide case study material which comprised specific information about key organizational changes they were in the process of implementing. Shortened descriptions of five of these case studies are included in this section to highlight what changes were perceived as priorities, why general managers valued the implementation of these changes and how the process of change was undertaken.

Four of the case studies (case studies 1–4) concern UGMs and one concerns a DGM (case study 5). As an illustration of the interplay between general managers' perceptions, values and behaviour in understanding the dynamics of organizational change, the case studies provide a number of insights. The case-studies were derived from interviews with general managers in the two years following implementation of the Griffith report. The cases are presented here in the present tense.

Case study 1: 'Re-locating psychiatric patients into the community'

Male UGM   Age 39
Job title   Unit General Manager, Psychiatric Services
Previous job title Director of Nursing Services
Scope of unit   Psychiatric Services [900 Beds]

1. Focus of change

The Regional Health Authority's policy is to secure relocation of large numbers of psychiatric patients into the community within a relatively shorter timescale. The UGM's intention was to achieve the Health Authority's policy by initiating the process of rehabilitation by returning psychiatric patients back into the community. Within this unit of 900 beds, the priority change was to re-accommodate all patients under 75 years of age with less than 20 years' stay by the year 1996.

Prior to his appointment in March 1986, the UGM considered that the unit's approach to community care was characterized by indecision and a lack of a clear policy of action despite the presence of a strategic plan. As a reaction to this vacill-ation, the objectives of the UGM's planned programme of change were clearly defined. Briefly, two main objectives were outlined: these were the closure of a large psychiatric hospital and the development of community psychiatric services. This commitment to community care was a major change in emphasis and would necessitate introducing a new management structure, changing staff attitudes to the community concept, developing appropriate facilities within the community, and improving public awareness of psychiatric services.

The UGM was extremely committed to this plan of change since he considered that the traditional pattern of psychiatric care was not only an ineffective use of public money but also resulted in the dehumanization of patients and restrictive staff practices. However, he was also aware that many of the unit's staff had a high tolerance of the *status quo* and corresponding negative attitudes to the concept of community care. It was apparent that the UGM's commitment to stop the 'warehousing' of psychiatric patients would require a massive reorganization in which the co-operation of staff at all levels was fundamental. Not only was this co-operation lacking, particularly from nurses and consultant medical staff, but financial constraints and shortage of time made the task even more daunting. In the face of these factors the UGM decided to initiate a 'high-profile' change strategy.

2. The change process

Soon after his appointment, the UGM was becoming increasingly aware of the lack of any agreed policy on community psychiatric care. As a consequence of this range of divergent views, the UGM decided to re-examine the issues of community care in a systematic manner and drew up a policy document outlining how to achieve the desired objectives. The UGM had made the restructuring of the unit's management an early priority, paying particular attention to the posts within the new structure.

In order to open up the debate about these issues and to explore the implications of the new policy, the UGM arranged a series of discussions with a wide range of individuals and groups within the district. In this attempt to gauge commitment whilst establishing a firm base from which to proceed, it became apparent that the tension and uncertainty which was rife amongst middle management, especially nurses, was counterbalanced by a groundswell of interest in community care emanating from junior staff. In an attempt to counter opposition to his proposals, the UGM exploited every opportunity to increase his visibility and the credibility of his plan by exposure and discussion with staff at all levels in the unit.

3. Perceived progress to date

The UGM feels that extensive discussion and debate is beginning to reduce the not insignificant opposition from nurses and consultant medical staff, but in retrospect he feels it would have been preferable and also have facilitated the change process if all staff had been allowed more time to discuss and explore the consequences and implications of the new initiatives.

In particular he now feels that he underestimated both the power of vested interest groups and the level of opposition he would encounter. Consequently he is now more aware of the importance of making small incremental steps to increase acceptance and credibility of any proposed change programme.

However, despite these difficulties, the UGM has secured a redundant school health clinic for conversion to patient accommodation. He has set dates for transferring some patients to this community abode and sees the achievement of this as a visible symbol of his determination to achieve the unit's objectives.

Links with the local authority housing bodies and voluntary associations (such as MIND) have been forged and these external groups appear to be supportive of his plans for community care.

The UGM intends to build on these initial successes in order gradually to secure the vital co-operation he requires and intends, over the next year, to develop additional bases for community psychiatric nurses to operate whilst extending his efforts to promote effectively his proposals for change.

4. Change evaluation checklist – graphical summary

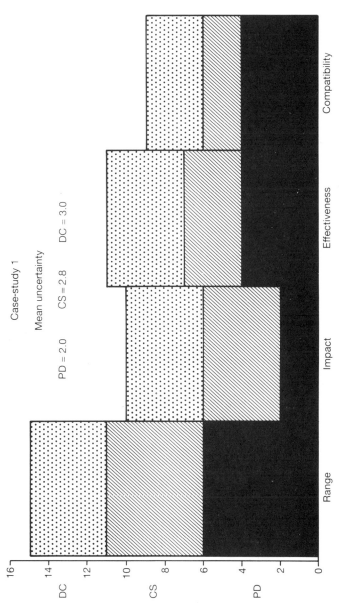

Figure 7.1 Graphical summary of change evaluation checklist for case-study 1.

Case-study 2: 'Encouraging clinicians to participate in the process of management'

Male UGM   Age 36
Job title   Unit General Manager, General/Obstetric
Previous job title Director of Planning and Administration
Scope of unit   General/Obstetric

1. Focus of change

The UGM was concerned with and recognized the vital contribution of clinicians to health care and firmly believed that the fundamental relationship in the NHS is that between doctor and patient. Since he considered that general management should embrace the providers of care, his key objective was to create an environment where the clinical contribution is allowed to flourish. His aim was to involve clinicians in a positive way in the process of management and anticipated that this would benefit the whole unit by helping him meet his objectives whilst ensuring a good working environment.

However, the UGM was fully aware that the medical professions have historically been critical of management, typically targeting their complaints on management's lack of commitment to patient care, lack of adequate communications and involvement and above all on management's unfair expectation that clinicians will 'pick up the pieces' generated by inadequate or inappropriate decisions. This negative attitude to management has often resulted in clinicians adopting a reactive role to management policy.

The UGM perceived the advent of general management as an ideal opportunity to develop co-operation and proactive medical involvement thus enabling some of the vital, but from the medical perspective less palatable, longer-term aspects of general management to be tackled. These issues include reductions in waiting lists and the measurement of clinical care.

More immediately, the acute unit (which comprises two main hospitals) needed to make overall financial savings in order to allow the service to expand. This, of course, would require considerable managerial skill, and in order for the UGM to make sound decisions he felt he must have access to the best available information. The UGM considers that the professional medical input is vital to the effectiveness of the decision-making process.

2. The change process

The initial catalyst for change occurred when the opportunity arose for the UGM to consider medical representation for the unit. At the first medical staff meeting he had attended, the UGM backed the medical proposal for two rather than one medical representative, and by this act reassured the clinicians that Griffiths-style management could operate in their interests. Despite the fact there was no expectation for regular attendance, the UGM continues to attend both medical staff committees at the two main hospitals.

In a similar confidence-building exercise, at an early stage in his job, the UGM declared his willingness to meet clinicians at their convenience in order to create a direct interface for discussion.

The UGM had individual discussions with the divisional chairman and all senior and middle managers, as well as with clinicians, and found a general receptiveness to his objectives. In this climate of increasing goodwill the UGM took the opportunity to begin to involve clinicians directly in the management process through joint medical/managerial involvement on specific issues of concern.

3. Perceived progress to date

The UGM currently meets the two medical representatives on a fortnightly basis and the UGM believes that this teamwork will grow as they get to know and understand each other better. Already he is aware of a shift in their style of involvement from passive implementation to active identification of issues that they wish to handle on his behalf. The willingness to become involved in the management process necessitates that medics maintain a certain independence between the demands of management on one hand and the expectations of their clinicial colleagues on the other. Maintaining a balanced perspective is something which the UGM considers he has also learned the value of and he recognizes that a certain detachment is required particularly if the medical viewpoint needs to be challenged. He considers this balance helps maintain his credibility and effectiveness in the face of competing demands.

The UGM feels that over the past year he has initiated the process of change, but securing the involvement of all clinicians in the process of management will take some considerable time. However, his view is that he is building a bridge to the future in which management will respect the medical profession's unique contribution to patient care and clinicians will respect management's ability to get things done.

4. Change evaluation checklist – graphical summary (see Figure 7.2)

Case-Study 3: 'Developing community-based services for the mentally handicapped'

Female UGM　　　　Age 34
Job Title　　　　Unit General Manager, Community/Mental Handicap
Previous Job Title　Director of Nursing Services, Primary Health Care
Scope of unit　　　Community/Mental Handicap and other District Services

1. Focus of change

The long-standing national commitment to the naturalization of certain patients is reflected in the Regional Health Authority's strategy to support the closure of some hospitals and to relocate many mentally-handicapped patients into the community. This strategy is based on the belief, shared by both the UGM and her DGM, that mentally-handicapped individuals, other than those with acute mental need, can enjoy a better quality of

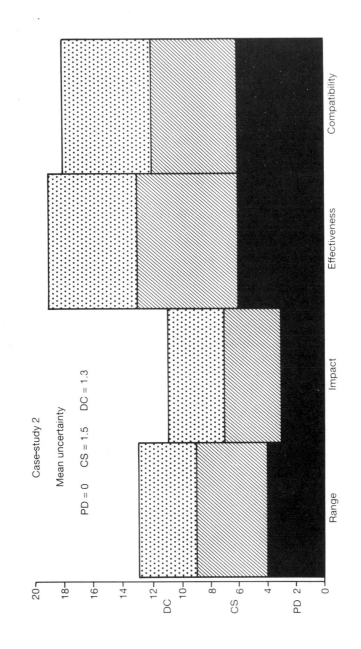

Figure 7.2 Graphical summary of change evaluation checklist for case-study 2.

life in the community than has been available to them in an institution.

Within this authority, the re-housing of patients is to be implemented through a joint health and social services document initiated since the appointment of the UGM in January 1986. Specifically, it is intended that by 1991 the new service will provide a range of small staffed homes for the mentally handicapped currently in hospital residence. In addition a small (ten-bed) in-patient facility is planned for those with severe disorders who require constant care.

The UGM considered that tackling this issue was a priority, since the advent of the new general management ethos offered an ideal opportunity to overcome the previous problems of diffuse authority and responsibility which were a characteristic of the old consensus arrangements. On a personal level the issue enabled the UGM to link her own appointment with a desirable visible improvement in provision for patient care. However, she is well aware that the medical staff within the mental handicap services feel justifiably threatened by the breadth of the proposed changes and she recognizes the need for their constructive involvement in order to minimize anxiety and uncertainty.

2. *The process of change*

On her appointment, the UGM was unhappy about the prevailing suggestion that a small (40-bed) mental handicap unit was to be pursued as part of the strategic plan, since she believed this would merely create a smaller institutionalized version of the current facilities, and this was not in the patients' best interests.

Acknowledging her concern, the DGM asked her to review the strategy and submit a proposal which better met the needs of patients. This proposal was discussed with the social services and a joint statement was produced which was made available to CHC, COHSE, NUPE and RCN staff for comments and constructive criticism. In April 1986 a joint statement of intent on mental handicap was signed by the DGM and the director of social services.

Following this joint statement, a joint group from the social and health services was set up to explore future options and this group met with professional and voluntary staff (including social workers, community workers, community nurses, MENCAP, and the league of friends) to discuss matters arising from the change proposals.

The next stage involved contacting housing associations in order to assess the availability of properties with respect to the financial and patient issues which their purchase might result in.

Further consultation and feedback involved the regional steering group, a university academic and a number of MPs who all provided comments, and as a result the cumulative final proposals were submitted to a panel for final agreement.

3. *Perceived progress to date*

Part of the hospital estate has been sold to help fund the changes and a number of community properties have been secured through a variety of channels, with staffing provided by the social services in some instances. A great deal of background work has resulted in the provision of an 'up-and-running' supporting structure to facilitate changes. This has included the development of the mental health register to provide better information on patients, examination of current facilities, and the production of explanatory booklets and literature. It is intended to appoint a joint project officer who will liaise between the health and social services and be responsible to the UGM, who, it is anticipated, will facilitate the change programme.

The UGM considers that the primary success of her first year in post has been the speed with which two authorities with different funding and cultures have produced a united joint approach. This co-operation is particularly signficiant since it will enable other aspects of the community services to be tackled in a joint fashion in the future.

However, the UGM's role embraces community services as well as mental handicap services and although she considers the effort put into the development of the new mental handicap strategy to be time well spent, she is aware that she has neglected the community aspect of her job. This has entailed the UGM adopting a reactive role and subordinates in the community services have been left to rely on their initiative; this is a situation with which understandably the UGM is less than happy.

4. Change evaluation checklist – graphical summary

Case-study 4: 'Reorganizing the structure of nursing management'

Male UGM	Age 46
Job Title	Unit General Manager, Community Unit
Previous Job Title	General Practitioner
Scope of unit	Community Services

1. Focus of change

The Regional Health Authority required the UGM to create a slimmer management structure for the community unit which as well as saving money would be more flexible in its operation. The UGM was keen for action in getting the unit on the road to becoming a better and more cost-effective service and he saw the new general managment ethos as providing a useful vehicle for implementing change. The UGM was particularly conscious that the public's perception of the community unit was vague and ill defined and he saw a primary goal in raising the profile of the community unit to match that enjoyed by the large hospitals.

Prior to the implementation of general management the UGM considered that there was considerable tension and inefficiency in the unit stemming from a previous 'traumatic' modification of nursing-management structures. However, the role of nurse management was still questionable and it was perceived to require redefinition and reorganization, although the UGM considered the district nursing and health visitor elements to have a number of strengths. There was a perceived skills gap for a number

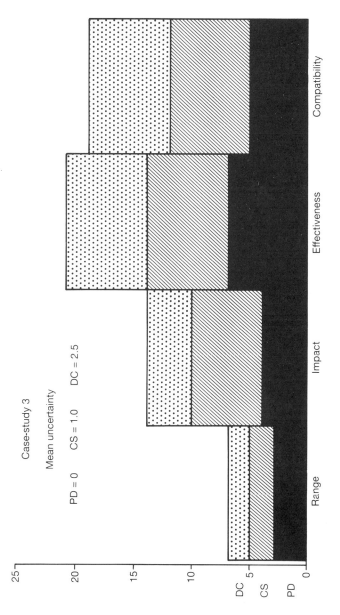

Figure 7.3 Graphical summary of change evaluation checklist for case-study 3.

of nurses who were not considered to have appropriate managerial skills.

2. The process of change

The DHA, although initially not enthusiastic for change, were required to conform to a national and regional initiative and they quickly moved from defending the *status quo* to strongly advocating innovation. The DHA required the UGM to produce a document defining and expanding his key objectives. The UGM's original proposal was to restructure nurses' management by creating two specialist systems for nursing and health visiting. However, following discussion with the DGM and a working party, changes were suggested to his original idea.

Instead of two specialist systems, a single generic structure was considered more appropriate; this would require the current three-tier arrangements being amalgamated into one unit. This proposal was followed by a six-week period of across-the-board consultation in which the nurses voiced a great deal of criticism. Their main concern focused on the reduction in the number of nursing posts, and the potential damage the changes would have on health visiting and district nursing as professions.

This period was characterized by much emotional turbulence coupled with a growing suspicion of the UGM's objectives. The UGM reports that during this period he realized the extent of his power and personal responsibility.

The next change involved filling the posts in the new management structure and some of the key posts were filled with internal appointments and other posts taken up by 'new blood' outsiders who were considered critical in enhancing the change and ensuring a balance in the new structure.

3. Perceived progress to date

The majority of the new appointments have now been taken up with the exception of the Unit Personnel Officer. The Unit Nursing Officer post was filled in September 1985 and influenced the filling of certain other key posts.

The UGM's desire to deal properly with existing employees whilst attempting to encourage 'new blood' into the unit has resulted in a number of temporary appointments which the UGM feels has inhibited progress on certain fronts.

In retrospect, the UGM considers that the short timescale for change set by the DHA did not give him enough time for general discussion or to study the system in detail before it was necessary for him to make decisions. This time shortage coupled with severe financial constraints constituted a significant pitfall for the UGM and generated a great deal of tension in attempting to draw up the new managerial structures. This tension was particularly manifested among the nursing profession and was exacerbated by existing senior nurse managers not succeeding in appointments within the new structure. The UGM acknowledges that he underestimated the resistance to change he encountered and now would have preferred to have built more flexibility into the new nurse management structure.

However, despite these difficulties, he feels that the process of review will give him the opportunity to take stock of the situation and initiate appropriate changes.

Change evaluation checklist – graphical summary

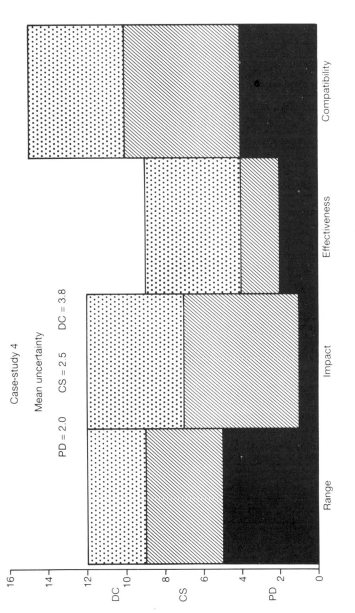

Figure 7.4 Graphical summary of change evaluation checklist for case-study 4.

Case study 5: 'Creating a health-orientated organizational culture'

Male DGM	Age 41
Job Title	District General Manager
Previous job title	District Administrator
Scope of district	Population – 250,000. Budget – £30 m

1. Focus of change

The DGM considers that the district is currently failing to provide for the needs of its population, and there is no likelihood of additional resources, although the current budget reflects the district's deprived social status. Within the district, the medical profession's opinion is that the rising pressure to provide medical treatment is due not only to the insatiable demands for 'cures' but also to the population's lack of attention in ensuring their own well-being. Consequently, the proposal for change is to curtail the organization's consumer-oriented approach, where the emphasis is placed on curing illness on a reactive basis, to a health-oriented approach where the emphasis centres on personal health care and the prevention of illness through the process of health education.

The attraction of this re-orientation is that it may divert some of the demand away from the acute sectors thereby releasing resources which can be used in other priority areas of health care.

The DGM has secured funding for additional staff to assist in this process of health promotion, but considers that those currently and intimately involved with patient care are best equipped to encourage users of the service to re-examine their lifestyles.

The general management ethos has created an innovative environment and the DGM feels that engendering the new culture is a bold attempt to instigate necessary changes. In contrast to the region's health promotion campaign which rests heavily on using the mass media, this approach is a localized strategy using what the DGM considers to be the health authority's biggest resource, its staff.

2. The process of change

Approximately 18 months ago a health promotion advisory group was set up chaired by the Senior Clinical Medical Officer. The group's key objective was to include those people who had a contribution to make and clinicians were involved to ensure that issues of patient care were taken into account. This group reports to the DHA annually and offers direction for the district policy group (previously the DMT).

The advisory group has adopted a 'bottom-up' approach and has actively sought opportunities to deliver its health promotional message to those directly involved in patient care. This is aimed at raising the profile of GP's by emphasizing the importance of co-operation between them and other community staff.

Although clinicians have a key role in the successful implementation of the new strategy, they have not, as yet, shown great enthusiasm for the new approach. The DGM feels that this lack of commitment is to be expected but anticipates that they will be persuaded of the values of the new approach over time if they are given continual exposure to its philosophy and on-going achievements.

3. Perceived progress to date

At the present time, the DGM considers that the authority is at the beginning of the transition stage and the completion date for change will not be evident for some time.

He has become very aware of the political dimensions surrounding the change issue and recognizes the need positively to involve clinicians in this process of cultural change. Specifically, the DGM is looking to the health promotion advisory group to prioritize specific targets in order to achieve an early success which can be subsequently built on. Evaluating and measuring these change interventions is perceived as being vital in convincing sceptics who are dubious of the value of the new approach.

The DGM feels that the achievement of a clear strategy about health promotion at the district level will now require the vehicle of UGM's involvement to deliver the services as close as possible to the consumer. 'Flatter' structures within units have been specifically designed to ensure maximum patient contact and the job descriptions of unit staff have been redesigned to take this additional responsibility into account.

In the movement from an 'illness-orientated' to a 'health-orientated' culture, the DGM anticipates that there will need to be a sustained momentum for change which will require careful handling by general management. Ultimately he feels a milestone will have been reached when the new philosophy is ingrained in all staff's approach to patient contact.

4. Change evaluation checklist – graphical summary (see Figure 7.5)

Common themes

It is apparent from the application of the checklist to these case studies that there appears to be a number of clear differences in the type and adequacy of these programmes of organizational change. However, despite these varying patterns inherent in the implementation of the change process, three common themes are evident in these examples of change and these are briefly identified below.

Firstly, it is apparent that all the general managers in the case studies saw the new general ethos as providing both an opportunity and a means of achieving organizational changes to which they were strongly committed. (The idea of general management as a 'vehicle' for the delivery of change was frequently expressed.) They were all of the opinion that, prior to their appointment, a sense of direction and a 'will' to change were often lacking;

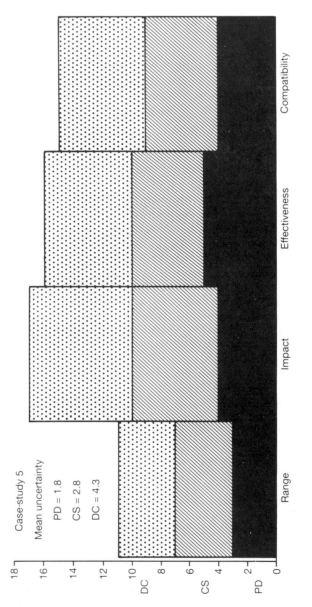

Figure 7.5 Graphical summary of change evaluation checklist for case-study 5.

this was reflected and reinforced by indecision, unclear objectives and often inefficiency and environments not conducive to effective working. Commitment to the new general management 'ethos' was strong and the general managers felt that the power and authority vested in their posts would enable them to 'get something done'. This optimism in the new order is clearly evident despite the apparently conflicting expectation that they should deliver a health service that is simultaneously better and more cost effective.

The second theme which permeates the case studies is the negative attitude to management displayed by the medical profession and nursing staff. This resistance to change was often expected but its strength was sometimes underestimated. Medical opposition to change was manifested in varying degrees across the case studies and the power of vested interest groups to either inhibit or facilitate the process of organizational change is clearly demonstrated. The desire of general managers to obtain the positive support and active involvement of clinicians in their proposals was apparent in all the case studies, although some general managers were initially more sensitive to the necessity of securing clinical co-operation.

The third issue which emerges from the case studies is the speed with which most changes were initiated and put on the path to full implementation. The pressure on general managers to effect rapid organizational change stems from a number of sources. The desire rapidly to rectify perceived organizational problems is augmented by short-term contracts and the expectation of others for visible signs of the new culture.

The necessity of initiating change as speedily as possible was seen as a challenge by some general managers and, in retrospect, a pitfall for others. This latter group was keenly aware of the lack of time in which fully to consult with colleagues and would have preferred more 'thinking time' before making key decisions which would result in major organizational upheaval. The case studies show that the boundaries between management by consensus and management by co-operation are still vague and ill defined in some quarters, and despite the formal power invested in the general management structure, the continuity of the traditional NHS culture continues to support the informal power of the medical interest groups. Reconciling the old with the new order is a major challenge for general management in this period of organizational transition.

CHAPTER 8
Investigating the implementation of general management

Background to the investigation

In previous chapters we have seen that the magnitude of changes with which a general manager is concerned can practically range from small-scale innovations such as re-designing an administrative system to large-scale changes such as overseeing the closure of hospitals. As the effects of the changes unfold, there has been a heightened awareness that their considerable impact and influence must be realistically assessed. It is too early yet to assess the outcome of some of these changes. However, it is not too early to consider the performance and progress of general managers in striving toward these objectives.

It has often been claimed that the essence of effective management is the management of change. Effective managers are those who are able to create, adopt and cope with organizational change. This process seems to involve matching the organization's structure and strategic response to both the environmental demands and the organization's innovatory capability. The issue of this 'matching' or compatibility of management's change strategies and effectiveness has been described in the previous chapters where it has been suggested that general managers' approaches are guided by their mental models of the organization.

In addition to stressing the structural and strategic components of the organization, we also contend that the success of a general manager in implementing organizational change will ultimately rest on his or her ability actively to shape the ideas and aspirations of the people in the system.

Of course, the various approaches to change need not be seen as mutually exclusive but more as different ways of approaching the proposed innovations. Macro-models which emphasize organizational structure, settings and contexts ultimately rest on the micro-models which emphasize attitudes, values and actions. From this perspective, the structure of an organization may be considered to rest on the cognitive (mental) models of its members. If the NHS is to change then the overt and covert behaviour of its members must also change.

In order to change the organizational structure and culture of the NHS a manager must ensure that both organizational and individual levels are considered as interacting components of the organization. This is necessary so that a clear unifying 'vision' is provided. This vision must highlight the new organizational goals and purposes whilst striving to inculcate the new beliefs and values which are required to support and facilitate the new initiatives for change.

Consequently, if we are to understand the process by which a general manager implements change we need to understand how he or she perceives the organization as it is at the present and how he considers it will develop under his/her management. This emphasis on examining how general managers view the structural, cultural and strategic factors which characterize their districts or units is the starting-point adopted in this study. By focusing on the internal mental models which general managers use as 'lenses' through which the organization is viewed, it becomes possible subsequently to examine their managerial activities with respect to their values and intentions. Tackling the 'values' issue is of critical importance in any cognitively-based approach since values provide the link between perceptions (i.e. how the organization is construed) and behaviour (i.e. what activities managers choose to perform).

The review of the literature on general management and organizational change (see Chapters 2 and 4) has highlighted the importance of distinguishing between what managers do (i.e. their actual behaviour and activities) and what managers intend to 'achieve' (i.e. their objectives and intended outcomes). Hales (1986) has convincingly argued that this is an important distinction which is often overlooked. Understanding the implications of this distinction is not merely a semantic exercise, since it is only through clearly distinguishing the performance from the expectation aspect of managerial work that it becomes possible to clarify what constitutes 'good' or 'bad' managerial practice.

The previous chapter has discussed several case studies of change and examined the reasons and rationale which general managers hold in support of the changes they had attempted to implement. This has provided a view of the change process in which managerial perceptions of organizational dynamics is crucial in understanding planned programmes of change.

By specifically examining perceptions of organizational change and preferred work activities, the aim of the study reported in this chapter is to present a coherent cognitively based account of the change strategies of general managers and to suggest how these results may be used in developing a measure for assessing their performance and progress.

The sample of participating managers

During 1987–88 a random sample of 100 NHS district and unit general managers were contacted by letter and asked to complete a 'kit' of measures relating to their perceptions of organizational change, preferred work activities, and specific organizational changes currently under way or 'in the pipeline'. Fifty-five general managers (46 UGMs and 9 DGMs) completed the exercise and this group forms the sample on which this study is based. The sample comprised 45 men and 10 women whose ages ranged from 30 to 60 years (average age, 41 years) only three of whom had been recruited outside the Health Service.

The measures used in the investigation

Two measures had been specifically developed for the purposes of this study. These have been called the Perception of Organizational Change Scale (POCS) and the Managerial Activities Questionnaire (MAQ). A copy of each measure together with its instructions for completion is included in the appendix. The construction, development and results obtained for each measure are discussed in turn. In this chapter work with the POCS is described and in Chapter 9 the results of the MAQ are presented and discussed.

Perception of organizational change scale (POCS)

The constituent items of the scale were carefully constructed bearing in mind three criteria. The items were intended to be

1. Representative – i.e. encompassing a wide range of change-related features
2. Relevant   – i.e. appropriate to general managers as agents of change in the NHS

and
3. Reliable   – i.e. unambiguous in their meaning for each respondent

The representativeness of the items in the scale was partially achieved by including a sufficiently large sample of items. However, size *per se* is not necessarily a virtue and needs to be balanced against respondent completion time. It would have been unreasonable to expect a busy general manager to spend an excessive amount of time completing an over-elaborate questionnaire, particularly when he was also required to complete the other measures which were included in the 'kit' sent to him.

Consequently, the POCS was restricted to 18 items relating to those general features of organizational change which had been highlighted in our examination of the literature and our studies of organizational change. The scale items which have been included are designed to tap managers' perceptions relating to organizational structure, managerial control, managerial problem-solving, attitudes to change, communication, performance criteria and reactions to change. These areas were those considered to be particularly relevant to understanding how general managers' perceive and think about the processes of organizational change.

The derivation of items from previous studies enabled a framework of analysis to be superimposed onto general managers' responses and their approaches to be subsequently classified and compared. In order to facilitate this comparison, the POCS was designed to contain two types of item: nine items concerned with managerial responsiveness to change and nine items referring to managerial control. The focus of these two types of item is itemized below.

Managerial responsiveness items

1. Extent of responsiveness to externally induced change

5. Extent of identification and assessment of significant organizational changes
6. Extent of dependence of problem-solving on emerging needs of the organization
7. Extent of acceptance and facilitation of managers to proposed organizational change
9. Extent of perceived frequency of external change which affects the stability of the organization
12. Extent of novel organizational problem-solving
13. Extent of performance standards reflecting novel innovatory criteria
17. Extent of the ability of the organization to anticipate future change
18. Extent of emphasis on ensuring continuity with past structures and practices.

Managerial control items

2. Extent of reliance on setting objectives and planning as methods of organizational control
3. Extent of changeability of internal organizational structure
4. Extent of reliance on written policies and procedures as methods of organizational control
8. Extent of formal power to implement organizational change
10. Extent of planning internal organizational structure
11. Extent of reliance on financial monitoring as methods of organizational control
14. Extent of reliance on formal communication channels for important information
15. Extent of external focusing of management efforts
16. Extent of freedom for individual members of the organization to structure their own jobs.

Piloting earlier versions of the POCS with NHS personnel had enabled ambiguities in the items to be identified and removed, thus ensuring their meaning to be as consistent as possible to different respondents.

Each of the eighteen items in the POCS has two parts.

(a) The first part of the item relates to that part of the organization for which the general manager has direct responsibility (i.e. a district or unit).
(b) The second part of the item relates to the organization as a whole (i.e. the NHS in general).

The general managers were required to rate parts (a) and (b) under each of the following three conditions:–

(i) **Present** – How they perceived the organization at the present time.
(ii) **Future** – how they thought the organization was likely to be in three years' time.
(iii) **Preferred** – How they would prefer the organization to be in three years' time.

It was stressed in the instructions that there were no right or wrong answers. The managers were required to mark each of the rating lines at the point which best represented their opinion. The ends of each 'rating line' were labelled and represent the point at which only one end of a dimension applies (see Appendix).

Scoring and analyzing the POCS

When completing each part of an item in the rating scale, general managers had the freedom to place a cross anywhere along each 'rating line' at the point which they considered best represented their opinion along a continuum between the item poles. In order to convert these ratings to scores which could be manipulated statistically, a seven-point template was used to superimpose on each rating line, so that each opinion point could be allocated a score from 1 to 7.

The structure of the POCS enabled the following sets of data to be compared for each of the items.

PART	A) Present	– GM's part of the organization
	B) Future	– GM's part of the organization
	C) Future preferred	– GM's part of the organization
WHOLE	D) Present	– Organization as a whole
	E) Future	– Organization as a whole
	F) Future preferred	– Organization as a whole

This structure enabled the general managers' perceptions of their own units and districts to be compared with their perceptions of the wider organization. Three types of measure of organizational change can be derived from the structure of the rating scale and these are described below.

1. **Expected change**

   By comparing general managers' perceptions of the present and future organization it was possible to determine how they expected the units or districts they manage to change over the next three years. Similarly by comparing perceptions of the wider organization at present and in the future, the general managers' expectations of change for the whole organization could be determined.

2. **Preferred change**

   By comparing general managers' perceptions of the organization at present and their future preferences, it was possible to determine their 'Preferred change – part' and their 'Preferred change – whole'.

3. **Future change deficiency**

   By comparing general managers' perceptions of the future organization and their preferred future changes, it was possible to examine the amount of deficiency or shortfall between changes they actually anticipate and changes they would prefer. In a sense, this comparison reflects the general manager's optimism about the innovatory potential of his or her own unit or district ('Future change deficiency – part') and for the organization as a whole ('Future change deficiency – whole').

The underlying structure of general managers' perceptions

It is clear that objective organization 'reality' is always viewed through the interpretive 'lens' of the general manager's subjective internal mental model. Managers may use many different descriptors to identify and understand organizational change but these descriptors are not all used independently. For example, a manager may consider that an 'inefficient' organization is generally also 'ineffective' and 'unresponsive'. In other words, managers expect one attribute to be associated or correlated with others. The pattern of these expected associations depends upon the way in which the manager thinks about the organization.

In order to examine whether general managers' perceptions of change could be usefully summarized and simplified, the ratings of all the managers in the sample were factor analyzed. Despite its mathematical complexity, the factor analysis technique is conceptually simple. No attempt is made here to tackle the underlying mathematics of the technique and the reader is referred to Harman (1967) for a detailed discussion.

There are various methods of factor analysis but most approaches start from calculating the correlation coefficients between every pair of items. This matrix of intercorrelations is then mathematically transformed in order to partition the items into separate sets of items which are then labelled as 'factors'. One of the primary aims of factor analysis is to summarize as much of the original information as possible. This is accomplished in the first extraction stage – where the correlations are resolved into a smaller number of underlying factors. In the second factor rotation stage, the factors which have been identified are mathematically 'rotated' in order to determine the simplest underlying structure which represents the best fit to the data.

The primary aims of factor analysis are data reduction and simplification and these objectives are applicable to the issue of attempting to examine the underlying structure in the POCS results. Our aim was to examine which items of the POCS tended to 'hang together' for the general manager group as a whole. Consequently, for each of the six rating conditions the factor analytic methods of principal components extraction and varimax rotation were applied to the data, resulting in six factor solutions.

Despite differences in factor solutions between rating conditions, it was evident that there were four common factors which occurred across all of the rating conditions. These common factors are listed below.

Factor A: Management planning and control
Factor B: Responsiveness to change
Factor C: Discontinuity with past procedures
Factor D: Flexibility of organizational structures.

These four common factors which have been identified may reflect the group's core conceptual model of the organization. There are underlying patterns to the domain of general managers' perceptions of the organization but understandably this structure is dependent on which aspects of the organization general managers are rating.

Group perceptions of organizational change

The scores from the Perception of Organization Change Scale were subsequently analyzed in two main ways. As a first comparison, general managers' responses were compared between their part and the whole organization on all 18 items. For eight of the nine managerial responsiveness items, general managers broadly considered that their own parts of the organization are more responsive than the wider organization both now and in the future.

As an example of how to interpret the tables, examine item 11 in table 8.2. It can be seen from this table that general managers expect both their part of the organization and the organization as a whole to rely on greater financial monitoring as a means of organization control in the future. This follows because the symbol '*' occurs in the 'part-expected change' and 'whole-expected change' columns of the table. However, in the future general managers would prefer that this method of managerial control only significantly increase within their part of the organization and not within the wider organization. This follows because the symbol '*' is only included in the 'part-preferred' column and not in the 'whole-preferred' column of table 8.2. This may well reflect the devolution of greater financial control down to units. Since both the 'part-future deficiency' and 'whole-future deficiency' columns are unmarked for this item we can conclude that, as a group, general managers do not anticipate any future shortfalls in financial monitoring as a method of managerial control

Table 8.1 Managerial responsiveness and types of perceived change

E = Expected change P = Preferred change F = Future change deficiency

ITEM	DESCRIPTION AND DIRECTION	PART E	PART P	PART F	WHOLE E	WHOLE P	WHOLE F
1.	Greater responsiveness to externally induced change	*	*	*	*	*	*
5.	Better identification and assessment of significant organizational change	*	*		*	*	*
6.	Greater dependence of problem-solving on emerging needs of the organization	*	*		*	*	*
7.	Greater acceptance and facilitation of managers to proposed organizational change				*	*	*
9.	Reduced frequency of external change which affects the stability of the organization		*	*		*	*
12.	Greater extent of novel organizational problem-solving	*			*	*	*
13.	Performance standards reflecting more novel innovatory criteria	*	*	*	*	*	*
17.	Greater ability of the organization to anticipate future change	*	*	*	*	*	*
18.	Less emphasis on ensuring continuity with past structures and practices					*	

Table 8.2 Managerial control and types of perceived change

E = Expected change P = Preferred change F = Future change deficiency

ITEM	DESCRIPTION AND DIRECTION	PART			WHOLE		
		E	P	F	E	P	F
2.	Greater reliance on setting objectives and planning as methods of organizational control	*	*	*	*	*	*
3.	More changeable internal organizational structure		*			*	*
4.	Less reliance on written policies and procedures as methods of organizational control					*	*
8.	Greater formal power to implement organizational change		*		*		
10.	Greater degree of planning of internal organizational structure						
11.	Greater reliance on financial monitoring as methods of organizational control	*	*		*		
14.	Greater reliance on formal communication channels for important information		*			*	
15.	Greater external focusing of management efforts					*	
16.	Greater freedom for individual members of the organization to structure their own jobs		*			*	*

The differences in how general managers viewed the development of the organization enabled a number of conclusions about their perception of the change process to be drawn. These results are briefly discussed below.

Responsiveness and power to implement change

General managers expect a number of similar changes to occur for both their own units and districts and for the organization as a whole. Within three years, general managers expect that throughout the NHS organizational change will be better anticipated, identified, assessed and responded to (see items 1, 5 and 17 in table 8.1). This increased anticipation and responsiveness to change will be necessary as the general management group do not anticipate any parallel reduction in the frequency of externally induced changes which will affect the stability of either their own units or districts or the organization as a whole (see item 9 in table 8.1). Interestingly, they consider their own domains to be less susceptible to externally-induced destabilizing change compared with the susceptibility of the whole organization.

This interpretation is supported by other comparisons of items in the POCS. Despite general managers' view that both their part and the wider organization are becoming more responsive to externally-induced change, the general managers only expected 'management as a whole' to become more accepting and facilitating of organizational change (see item 7 in table 8.1). Paradoxically, they did not expect their own future attitudes and behaviour to become more accepting of innovation. The reasons for this discrepancy may be apparent when we examine another significant difference in managers' ratings. It is apparent that the managers felt that they currently are, and in the future would remain, significantly more accepting and facilitating of proposed change than management as a whole. It is clear that part of the general managers' self-concept is that they hold more positive attitudes to change than the rest of the NHS management, and they consequently consider that they have little scope for further increasing their acceptance and facilitation of organizational change. This perceived difference may be defensive and reflect the view that since they have been the champions of change, there is little further scope for taking further change initiatives on board.

The Griffiths Report had emphasized that consensus management and widespread consultation was responsible for a great deal of organizational inertia within the NHS. Consequently it is not surprising that general managers will meet resistance and negative attitudes which could undermine the effective management of change. This resistance will continue to operate as long as the many powerful interest groups in the NHS are unenthusiastic or antagonistic to the management reforms recommended by the Griffiths inquiry.

In the face of this resistance to innovation, it is understandable that general managers would prefer that they possessed greater formal power to ensure the implementation of their chosen programmes of organizational change. This is evident from an inspection of item 8 in table 8.2, although despite this preference, they did not actually expect any future increase in their level of formal power within the next three years. The NHS can be considered to comprise various interest groups whose power, interests and aspirations are not always compatible, and the dominant power group within the NHS has been the medical profession. The Griffiths inquiry, while recognizing the importance of doctors, proposed a different balance of power which questioned the medical profession's traditional dominance. Although many clinicians would argue that this new balance of power has gone too far in the direction of the general management ethos, our results indicate that general managers themselves would welcome even more power to implement change. Clearly, any proposed organizational change will affect the complex set of relationships which exist between the interest groups which comprise a district or unit and the response of these groups will depend to a large extent on how these proposed changes are perceived to serve their own interests. Consequently, the medical profession is and will continue to be extremely influential in either resisting or facilitating programmes of planned change.

If effective progress is to be made, proposed changes which stem from the new general management ethos should be effectively communicated and disseminated within the NHS. The diffusion of any innovative idea takes place as information is communicated through the appropriate social systems by the groups and individuals of which the organization is comprised. It can be seen from item 14 in table 8.2 that general managers would prefer that in future there should be greater reliance on formal communication channels for important information, not only within their own units or districts but in the organization as a whole. However, they do not expect the reliance on 'informal' or 'grapevine' communication significantly to diminish in the future.

As a group, general managers feel that their power to implement organizational change is curtailed, and this perceived 'powerlessness' is seen to result to some extent from the 'dilution' of their change interventions by the inertial effects of 'informal' interest groups and 'informal' communication.

Problem-solving and strategic planning

In addition to handling the political problems of internal interest groups, one of the essential capabilities of general management is to strike the right balance between ensuring sufficient momentum for change whilst maintaining on-going organizational control and efficiency. The structure of the POCS reflects these two contrasting objectives.

The results suggest that general managers believe that the NHS will become more reactive to the emerging needs of the organization with respect to problem-solving (see item 6 in table 8.1), and, in the future, managers believe that performance standards will be based on more novel innovatory criteria than they are at present (see item 13 in table 8.1).

In contrast to this greater reactivity, the managers also consider that in the future greater reliance will be placed in setting objectives and planning as methods of organizational control (see item 2 in table 8.2) and ideally they would like to see these approaches becoming even more important in the future. This recognition that NHS systems of planning are in need of some improvement was highlighted in the Griffiths report: 'There is no driving force seeking and accepting direct and personal responsibility for developing management plans, securing their implementation and monitoring actual achievement'

Rathwell (1986) has pointed out that the inability of current NHS planning systems to respond to the demands placed upon them is partly a function of the planning systems themselves and partly a consequence of the intrinsic managerial complexities of the NHS. The general manager has to cope with rapidly changing organizational, political, social and economic environments and in this turbulence, the role of planning becomes increasingly important as a means of increasing the visibility and predictability of future change. Applied appropriately, planning can be an important means of ensuring that the organization becomes less reactive and more anticipating and proactive in creating and coping with change.

General managers' anticipated and preferred direction of change reflects the movement away from management control systems relying on written policies and procedures toward a more strategically orientated planning approach in the future (see items 2 and 4 in table 8.2). However, general managers consider that, even after three years, this increased reliance on planning will not have become as important as they would ideally prefer. This expected organizational shift toward a more strategic planning approach will necessitate general managers making a series of trade-offs between choosing management strategies which are either continuous or discontinuous with past policies and procedures. The advantage of choosing strategies which are broadly continuous with the past is that this enables the positive transfer of the organization's capabilities and experience to the new change ventures. However, the advantage of selecting strategies which are discontinuous with the past is that a radically new approach may significantly enhance the possibility of significant organizational improvement. Clearly a radical discontinuous approach is riskier and often more difficult to implement than a broadly continuous approach, although its benefits may prove significantly greater.

It appears that general managers would like the organization as a whole to place less emphasis on ensuring continuity with the past organizational structures and practices, although they do not expect this change to take place within three years (see item 18 in table 8.1). However, they consider that their own units or districts have already become sufficiently discontinuous with the past and consequently do not need to proceed any further in this direction.

These results can be viewed in the context of organizational theory which frequently contends that different strategic approaches require different organizational capabilities. Continuous strategies generally require stable internal environments based on functional divisions of labour. In contrast, discontinuous strategies generally require the organization to be responsive to environmental pressure and capable of rapid effective organizational change. Within the NHS, the transition from functional to general management is paralleled by the general managers' perceived need for the organization as a whole to adopt a discontinuous strategic response to the demands of change. Unfortunately, they appear to be sceptical of this actually happening in the foreseeable future.

Preferred and expected changes

An examination of the results showed that there were a number of discrepancies between preferred and expected changes. It was apparent that nine of the general managers' preferred changes are expected to come to fruition within three years either for their part or for the whole organization; these were POCS items, 1, 2, 5, 6, 7, 11, 12, 13 and 17. In contrast there are seven preferred items which are not expected to occur within three years, neither for their part nor for the whole organization (see items 3, 4, 8, 9, 15, 16, and 18). There are clear differences beween the types of preferred changes which are expected to occur and the types of preferred changes which are not expected to occur. These differences are shown in table 8.3.

The items have been broadly categorized into four types and it is apparent that the preferred/expected changes are mainly of type 1, 'cultural awareness and responsiveness to change', whereas the preferred/not-expected changes are mainly of type 3, 'structurally-related changes'. Similarly, 'planning and budgeting as methods of organizational control' (type 2) are preferred and expected whereas 'less internal focusing and dependence on written policies and procedures' (type 4) are preferred but not expected.

Table 8.3 Preferred changes, expected and not expected

Preferred changes – expected to occur	Preferred changes – not expected to occur
1. Cultural awareness and responsiveness to change (Items 1, 5, 6, 7, 12, 13, 17)	3. Structurally-related changes (Items 3, 8, 16, 18)
2. Planning and budgeting as methods of organizational control (Items 2, 11)	4. Less internal focusing and dependence on written policies and procedures (Items 4, 15)

[Item 9, reduced frequency of destabilizing external conditions, is not included in any category type since it represents a preferred change over which management has little or no direct control.]

The reasons for these differences in change expectations are open to speculation, but they might reflect two factors which impinge on general managers' attempts to innovate. Firstly, for a variety of reasons the preferred/expected changes might be considered easier or quicker to achieve than those changes which are not expected to occur within three years. Secondly, general managers might consider that the preferred/expected changes have a higher priority than those changes which are not expected.

Future shortfalls in organizational change

One general theme which has run through this discussion of the items in the POCS is that general managers consider their own districts and units to be 'superior' to the organization as a whole with respect to a number of items. Tables 8.1 and 8.2 show that general managers think that the districts and units they are responsible for are currently and also will continue to be more responsive, less rigid and more innovative in their approach (see items 1, 2, 4, 5, 7, 12, 13 and 15) compared with the organization as a whole. However, general managers do not consider their own domains to be signficantly different from the wider organization with respect to those items reflecting flexibility and planning of organizational structure, power to implement change and ability to anticipate future changes (see items 3, 8, 10, 11, 14, 15 and 17).

Some light is thrown on these differences by examining the 'future change deficiencies' revealed in general managers' ratings. The future change deficiency measure is the difference between what general managers consider the actual future organization will be like compared with what they consider their preferred future organization ought to be like. Significant deficiencies or shortfalls are apparent for only four items relating to general managers' own organizational domains but for twelve items relating to the organization as a whole. In other words, general managers think that their own units or districts will become much closer to the future 'ideal' than the organization as a whole, and the rest of the organization has a great deal of 'catching up' to do in order to match their own level of perceived responsiveness, flexibility and innovation.

Broadly, it appears that general managers believe they have initiated and will continue to influence some cultural improvements and management control strategies within their own districts and units but appear less optimistic about engineering on-going structural changes or freeing themselves and their organizations from an over-emphasis on written policies and procedures. The picture of general management presented by the POCS is an uneasy mixture of short-term cultural optimism constrained by a pragmatic assessment of organizational continuity and inertia in a complex turbulent environment.

Group results of this kind can provide a broad overview of general managers' perceptions of organization change, but individual perceptions are also very important. In the next chapter we introduce a technique which is able to focus upon the activities and intentions of general managers and enables individual differences between managers to be examined in greater detail.

CHAPTER 9

Managerial activities and intentions

The purpose of this chapter is to explore the theme that the behaviour of general managers in tackling organizational change in the NHS needs to be viewed not only with respect to what is done but also with respect to how personal and organizational objectives are construed. In other words, the implementation of organizational change ultimately rests on how general managers perceive the nature of this change and their role in structuring their own personal and organizational objectives into appropriate activities.

Understanding the conceptual frameworks which underpin managerial activities could have profound implications for assessing the performance of general managers. As Hales (1986) has observed, the problem of much of the managerial research to date has been the reluctance to ask why managers behave in the way they do.

Consequently, if we are to understand the process by which a general manager implements change we need to understand how he perceives the organization as it is at the present and how he considers it will develop under his or her management. The previous chapter has examined how general managers view the structural, cultural and strategic factors which characterize their districts or units. By focusing on the internal mental models which general managers adhere to, it becomes possible subsequently to examine their managerial activities with respect to their values and intentions. Tackling the 'motives' issue is of critical importance in any cognitively-based approach since these intentions provide the link between perceptions (i.e. how the organization is construed) and behaviour (i.e. what activities managers choose to perform).

The activities of general management

We have seen in Chapter 2 that observational studies of managers' jobs have not really revealed any clearly-defined set of well-demarcated managerial activities. Although it seems reasonable to assume that most managers engage in a series of activities such as setting objectives, planning, organizing, communicating and monitoring, this neat structure has not been reflected in examination of what managers actually do in their jobs. The work of researchers like Mintzberg and Kotter has shown that most managerial behaviour does not conform to a neat package of functional stages. In fact, the picture of managers' work which is emerging is characterized by a pattern of disjointed 'juggling' of tasks where little time is spent on any activity in particular, but a great deal of time is spent in brief fragmented conversations with others. This frantic managerial 'fixing' takes place both inside and outside the organization and on the surface, at least, gives the impression of chaos and disorder. However, if a general manager's personal agenda for action and his communication networks are very well organized then brief bursts of purposeful conversation are an extremely effective means of accumulating a large volume of relevant information. It has been argued that the general manager is able to exercise his control and influence over others using this strategy coupled with bargaining and bartering for reciprocal 'good turns'. Whether this frenetic activity is 'good' management practice is yet to be resolved.

In a recent review of the evidence relating to what managers do in their jobs, Hales (1986) has identified a conceptual confusion between what managers 'do' (i.e. their actual behaviour and activities) and what managers intend to 'achieve' (i.e. their desired goals). In simple terms, what a manager does should be distinguished from the reasons for doing it. This is not merely a matter of semantics since there are important practical implications in attempting to clarify what constitutes 'good' or 'bad' managerial practice. Hales (1986) has suggested that progress in tackling the 'managerial effectiveness' issue should examine the relationship between performance and expectations.

In other words, effectiveness may be more to do with the 'appropriateness' of particular intentions in supporting particular activities and this is the approach we have adopted in the present chapter. Our belief is that managerial motives and activities should not be considered as separate areas, a view which was originally expressed by the distinguished psychologist P. G. Herbst (1970).

> The statement 'I act' may be separated into the 'I' that acts and the 'activity' . . . . Here it may be possible to be misled by the theory on which our conventional language is based. We say that 'the table has legs' and thus assert that there exists a table apart from the board and legs. The legs form part of the table. We say 'the lightning flashes' but the lightning and the flash are one and the same thing.

If we represent the person in terms of the activities he engages in, that is, we say the activities form part of the person, we arrive at the behaviour system concept. Motivation and emotions can then no longer be considered as belonging to a separate system which is linked to the behaviour, but have to be looked at as characteristics of a behaviour system.

The Managerial Activities Questionnaire (MAQ)

Despite the diversity in the types of managerial activities which researchers have proposed to date, there does appear to be a common set of activities which it seems reasonable to assume all managers engage in. Fifteen pairs of such common activities were identified for inclusion in the MAQ, which was developed in order to examine general managers' preferred activities and their associated intentions for their job behaviours. A copy of the original MAQ is shown in the Appendix, although another version has been subsequently developed with a simplified scoring system. A copy of this new version of the questionnaire , together with scoring instructions, is included later in this chapter to give the reader an opportunity to ascertain his or her own activity-intention style.

Each general manager in our sample (n = 55) was required to consider each pair of activities in turn and to choose their preferred activity from each pair. Two managers had not completed the questionnaire properly and results reported in this chapter are based on 53 respondents. Having selected their preferred activity, the managers were asked to give their reasons for choosing that activity or rejecting the other one. If they were unable to decide which activity they preferred, they were asked to explain why they liked or disliked both of them. It was stressed that there were no right or wrong answers and the managers were asked to avoid vague answers such as 'I like it', 'I prefer it' and so on.

By examining the reasons for each general manager's preferred activities it became possible to examine how the activities of mangement are construed and understood by managers. A similar comparison technique has been used in a previous measure (the 'Job Features Questionnaire', Bergwerk and Clarke, 1982) but unlike the MAQ this technique was directed at facilitating organizational selection and placement.

By asking general managers to state why they prefer some activities over others, we are investigating the criteria by which they judge their management activities and what they conceive as the relative advantages and disadvantages of their choices. One of the hallmarks of managerial work is that the manager is typically free to define his or her own job both in terms of what is done (the work content) and how it is to be done (the work method). Stewart (1982) has demonstrated and discussed the wide variety of ways in which managers perform what would appear nominally to be the same jobs. The MAQ separates what a general manager does from why he does it and the results which were obtained enable managerial activities and intentions to be examined simultaneously. In this way, it becomes possible to describe what managerial activities mean to managers in terms of their value to the manager.

Scoring the MAQ

General managers' reasons for choosing activities were coded into the twelve categories of intention shown below.

1. ES **Enjoyment/interest satisfaction – self**
   (i.e. It enhances my own enjoyment, interest or satisfaction)
2. EO **Enjoyment/interest/satisfaction – other**
   (i.e. It facilitates others' enjoyment, interest or satisfaction)
3. IS **Innovation/expansion/development – self**
   (i.e. It helps me expand my impact or be more innovative)
4. IO **Innovation/expansion/development – other**
   (i.e. It helps others expand their impact or be more innovative)
5. AS **Achieving aims/objectives/goals – self**
   (i.e. It helps me achieve my own personal aims, objectives or goals)
6. AO **Achieving aims/objectives/goals – other**
   (i.e. It helps others achieve their aims, objectives and goals)

  7. US **Utility/effectiveness/efficiency – self**
     (i.e. It enables me to be more effective or efficient)
  8. UO **Utility/effectiveness/efficiency – other**
     (i.e. It enables others to be more effective or efficient)
  9. RS **Role appropriateness/expectation/performance – self**
     (i.e. It enables me to fulfil the role expectations appropriately)
 10. RO **Role appropriateness/expectation/performance – other**
     (i.e. It enables others to fulfil the role expectations appropriately)
 11. PS **Power/control/understanding – self**
     (i.e. It enhances my own organizational understanding and influence)
 12. PO **Power/control/understanding – other**
     (i.e. It enhances others' organizational understanding and influence).

Categorizing general managers' activities and intentions in this way enables
comparisons to be made between managers in order to highlight what activities
mean to managers in terms of their motives and intentions. By assigning the
managers intentions for choosing an activity to a category scheme, it is possible
to examine the areas of discrepancy and interaction between their activities
and intentions, not only for the group as a whole, but for individual general
managers.

General managers' preferred activities and intentions

In completing the MAQ, the sample of general managers (n = 53) generated
a total of 1,256 intentions to support their choices of preferred managerial
activities. These reasons were coded in accordance with the twelve categories
described above and the frequencies cross-classified with the thirty managerial
activities (fifteen pairs) contained in the measure. Table 9.1 shows the
percentage frequencies of the general managers' choice of activities and each
activity's most frequently cited intentions. The preferred activities for all fifteen
pairs are those that appear in the top half of the table and the unpreferred
activities are those that appear in the bottom half of the table. Both activities
in pair number 6, 'Engaging in long-range strategic planning' v 'Engaging
in short-range opportunistic planning' received a 50% endorsement and consequently, activities above this pair in the table are those which the group
preferred and items below this pair in the table were those which were not
preferred.

   It can be seen from this table that as a group there is a strong consensus
of preferred work activities. These common choices reflect a strong shared
identity of what it means to be a general manager in the NHS, and can be
usefully related to what organizational changes general managers have selected
for their attention. These issues are tackled later in the chapter.

   What is particularly interesting is that different activities tend to be
supported by different patterns of intentions, although there is a strong current
of popular intentions running through all the managerial activities. Improving
organizational effectiveness (UO) and self-effectiveness (US) are the most
frequently cited intentions. Enhancing self enjoyment, interest or satisfaction
(ES) also ranks highly, in contrast to enhancing the enjoyment, interest

Table 9.1 MAQ choice of activities and associated most frequently cited intentions for the general manager sample (n = 53)

PAIR NO. MANAGERIAL ACTIVITIES	% FREQUENCY	MOST FREQUENTLY CITED INTENTIONS			
11. Allocating resources	100%	US	UO	AO	
15. Asking/persuading people to do things	98%	US	UO	ES	
12. Initiating innovating activities	96%	ES	RS	IS	IO
1. Expanding your contact network	94%	UO	US	IS	IO
7. Leading the organization	94%	RS	ES	US	
10. Dealing with matters requiring specialist expertise	90%	RS	RO	ES	
2. Making decisions	89%	UO	US	ES	
13. Reviewing subordinates progress	85%	UO	US		
14. Communicating with people not at your level in the organization	84%	US	UO	ES	
4. Dealing with strategic organizational issues	83%	RS	RO	ES	
8. Briefing subordinates	80%	RO	UO		
5. Participating in unplanned informal face-to-face meeting	79%	UO	US	ES	
9. Setting personal agendas for action	77%	US	UO	RS	RO
3. Disseminating information	71%	UO	US	ES	
6. Engaging in long-range strategic planning	50%	US	UO	ES	
6. Engaging in short-range 'opportunistic' planning	50%	US	UO	ES	
3. Receiving/monitoring information	29%	UO	US		
9. Controlling the organizational workflow	23%	RO			
5. Participating in planned formal meetings	21%	UO	US	ES	
8. Controlling/directing subordinates	20%	PO	UO		
4. Dealing with day-to-day organizational disturbances	17%	ES	AO	RO	
14. Communicating with people at your level in the organization	16%	ES	US	UO	
13. Setting your own job boundaries	15%	UO	US		
2. Implementing decisions	11%	ES	AO	RO	
10. Dealing with general administrative duties	10%	US			
7. Acting as a spokesman/figurehead for the organization	6%	RS			
1. Maintaining your contact network	6%	US	UO	ES	
12. Participating in advisory or negotiating activities	4%	US			
15. Telling/ordering people to do things	2%	ES			
11. Preserving assets	0%				

or satisfaction of others (EO) which was, sadly, rarely cited as a supporting intention. Ensuring role appropriateness for self and others (RS and RO) also ranks fairly highly and tends to occur across a range of activities. The percentage frequency and ranks for the twelve types of intention are shown in table 9.2.

Table 9.2 Percentage frequencies and ranks for the twelve categories of general managers' intentions (n = 53)

			PERCENTAGE	RANK
UO	Utility/Effectiveness/Efficiency	Other	19.64	1
US	Utility/Effectiveness/Efficiency	Self	17.86	2
ES	Enjoyment/Interest/Satisfaction	Self	15.36	3
RS	Role Appropriateness/Expectation/Awareness	Self	14.64	4
RO	Role Appropriateness/Expectation/Awareness	Other	9.38	5
IO	Innovation/Expansion/Development	Other	4.91	6
AO	Achieving Aims/Objectives/Goals	Other	4.55	7
PO	Power/Control/Understanding	Other	4.20	8
IS	Innovation/Expansion/Development	Self	4.02	9
AS	Achieving Aims/Objectives/Goals	Self	2.95	10
PS	Power/Control/Understanding	Self	1.61	11
EO	Enjoyment/Interest/Satisfaction	Other	0.89	12

As an example of the interaction between managerial activities and intentions, consider activity pair in table 9.1. Here, both the maintenance and expansion of a contact network were supported by the intentions of improving organizational effectiveness (UO and US) but whereas the least popular choice (maintaining contact network) was also frequently supported by the self enjoyment/interest category (ES), the most popular choice (expanding contact network) was frequently supported by the innovation categories (IS and IO). In other words, a small percentage of general managers prefer the personal enjoyment resulting from maintaining their established contacts whereas a much larger percentage of general managers prefer the innovatory potential of network expansion. Most of the general managers in this sample are new to the post, and this finding reflects Kotter's (1982) observations about the importance of network building particularly in the early term of office of general managers. Kotter has shown that the subsequent efficient implementation of an agenda (i.e. tasks to be achieved) rests on the prior development of a good contact network.

In a similar way, the interaction between activities and intentions can be examined for the remaining fourteen pairs of activities contained in the MAQ. These are briefly discussed below.

The vast majority of the general managers preferred making decisions rather than implementing them as they felt this to be the most efficient use of their time. However, several general managers preferred implementing decisions because they enjoyed 'getting involved'. Mintzberg (1973) has highlighted the importance of effective managers 'meddling in the activities of their staff' by being willing to tackle the problems of their subordinates although the desire to become involved with day-to-day organizational problems was shunned by most of the general managers. Typically they felt it was more role appropriate for both themselves and their subordinates that they focused their efforts on dealing with strategic organizational issues. For the same reason they over-whelmingly preferred dealing with matters requiring their specialist expertise rather than dealing with general administrative duties, although oddly perhaps, one or two considered general administration to be preferable. This could be an example of managers focusing on those activities which they know best and find intrinsically satisfying. Dimmock (1985) has pointed out that an absence of a general management tradition in the NHS may heighten the probability of some general managers falling back into established and comfortable patterns of work.

Although the majority of general managers recognized the importance of dealing with strategic organizational issues, they were, as a group, clearly divided on whether they preferred to engage in long-range strategic planning or short-range 'opportunistic' planning. Both contrasting activities were supported by the same pattern of intentions which reflected self and organiza-tional efficiency together with personal satisfaction. However, with respect to participating in meetings the majority felt that unplanned informal 'face-to-face' meetings were both more efficient and enjoyable than planned formal meetings, although these were preferred by some general managers for the same set of intentions.

This preference for the unplanned face-to-face meetings is in accordance with the interactive view of management described by Mintzberg (1973) and Kotter (1982). This perspective is further supported by the general managers' group preference for disseminating information over receiving or monitoring information and their majority preferences for setting personal action agendas and communicating with people at all levels in the organization. The general manager is in a central position for the assimilation and redistribution of information and Mintzberg (1973) has described the monitoring of information as an activity which enables a better understanding of events by 'intelli-gence gathering' rather than by studying formal reports. The dissemination of information involves transmitting information to subordinates which is not simply factual but contains guidelines and preferences. General managers' preference for the briefing rather than the monitoring component of Mintzberg's 'informational' role suggests that they are well aware of the value of active directed interaction.

As a group, the general managers preferred a participative rather than an authoritarian style, reflected in their preferences for briefing and persuading subordinates rather than directing or ordering them. They generally felt the participative style to be more pleasant and effective. Kotter (1982) found that the effective general manager relied more on requests and persuasion than intimidation to achieve objectives, and in Kotter's study general managers rarely issued orders. Kotters findings are confirmed in this study.

General managers clearly preferred the global activities of leading the organization and initiating innovations over acting as a 'figurehead' or negotiating. They considered the leadership and change agent roles as appropriate to their position and personally satisfying. These results are somewhat surprising since Mintzberg (1973) has identified acting as a 'figurehead' as a core function of senior managers. Similarly, the abilities of a general manager to negotiate would appear to be vitally important as Dimmock (1985) suggests, particularly with respect to the thorny issue of allocating resources. As Dimmock (1985) observes 'it seems likely that the new general managers will face their stiffest test when they begin negotiations with the powerful clinical interests'.

From these interactions it appears that the culture of general management is being expressed in the following ways.

1. There is a strong pressure to extend personal networks as a mechanism for implementing changes. This is in accord with the findings of Kotter (1982) and Stewart and Wyatt (1985).
2. Managers much prefer decision-making to the process of doing things. This more strategic orientation is part of the new general mangagement ethos.
3. There is a shift from prior concerns with administrative detail to most managers now wishing to direct their expertise into specialist or priority areas.
4. There is a marked preference for informal, face-to-face meetings. Again this is in accord with previous findings suggesting managers should devote their energy to receiving, communicating and disseminating information.

The analysis of activity/intention interactions in this way can prove valuable in two main ways. Firstly, it opens up the possibility of examining the appropriateness of what general managers consider their activities will achieve. The issue of appropriateness cannot be effectively resolved by considering managerial activities in isolation.

For example, several general managers preferred implementing rather than making decisions. This choice, although atypical, is not necessarily inappropriate, but could be indicative of ineffectiveness if supported by reasons of enjoying active participation in subordinates' tasks, since this might imply an inability to delegate. Concern with this potential failure was expressed by some general managers. Similarly, a small proportion of general managers preferred dealing with general administrative duties rather than applying their specialist expertise, since they were already proficient in this area through their previous experience in administration. Again this raises the issue of appropriateness. One general manager preferred to order rather than to ask or to persuade people to do things, not for reasons of greater efficiency, which arguably might be appropriate, but because he enjoyed exercising power over others. Consequently, the analysis of activity/intention interactions could prove potentially beneficial as a diagnositc device for managerial performance.

The second potential benefit from this form of analysis is that it might form the basis of a typology into which general managers could be classified. If a typology of activities and intentions is predictive of the ways in which general managers perceive and implement organizational change, then useful inroads could be made into the complex problem of assessing and comparing the progress and performance of general managers across a diverse range of health districts.

Some preliminary evidence towards this general goal is presented below.

General Managers activity types and motives

The MAQ comprises 30 managerial activities and these are considered to be subsumed under the four broad activity types (1–4) listed below.

Activity type 1 – liaising (8 MAQ activities)
Maintaining your contact network
Disseminating information
Participating in unplanned informal face-to-face meetings
Participating in advisory or negotiating activities
Reviewing subordinates progress
Communicating with people at your level in the organization
Communicating with people not at your level in the organization
Asking/persuading people to do things

Activity type 2 – planning (8 MAQ activities)
Expanding your contact network
Receiving/monitoring information
Participating in planned formal meetings
Engaging in long-range strategic planning
Engaging in short-range strategic planning
Setting personal agendas for action
Allocating resources
Setting your own job boundaries

Activity type 3 – implementing (7 MAQ activities)
Implementing decisions
Dealing with day-to-day organizational disturbances
Controlling/directing subordinates
Briefing subordinates
Controlling the organizational workflow
Dealing with general administrative duties
Initiating innovating activities

Activity type 4 – leading (7 MAQ activities)
Making decisions
Dealing with strategic organizational issues
Leading the organization
Acting as a spokesman/figurehead for the organization
Dealing with matters requiring specialist expertise
Preserving assets
Telling/ordering people to do things

Each reason general managers had suggested to support their activity choices had been previously coded into the twelve intention categories described earlier and these twelve categories were themselves further aggregated into the four types of motive (A–D) described.

Motive type (A)   Facilitating own task performance
Innovation/expansion/development	Self
Achieving aims/objectives/goals	Self
Utility/effectiveness/efficiency	Self

Motive type (B)   Facilitating others' task performance
Innovation/expansion/development	Other
Achieving aims/objectives/goals	Other
Utility/effectiveness/efficiency	Other

Motive type (C)   Enhancing own organizational role
Enjoyment/interest/satisfaction   Self
Role appropriateness/expectation/awareness   Self
Power/control/understanding   Self

Motive type (D)   Enhancing others' organizational role
Enjoyment/interest/satisfaction   Other
Role appropriateness/expectation/awareness   Other
Power/control/understanding   Other

All of the participating managers' responses on the MAQ were cross-categorized using these four activity-type categories together with the four motive-type categories to examine the distribution of the general managers' responses. It was clear that different managerial activity types are differentially associated with a different pattern of motives. These frequencies were converted into a weighted percentage for each of the 16 activity type/motive type combinations and these are shown in table 9.3. (The weighting was necessary since the activity types 'liaising' and 'planning' each comprised eight activities and the activity types 'implementing' and 'leading' each comprised seven activities).

Table 9.3   *Weighted percentage scores for each of the sixteen activity type/motive type categories*

| | | MOTIVE TYPES | | | | |
| | | FACILITATING | | ENHANCING | | |
		Own tasks	Others' tasks	Own role	Others' role	TOTAL ROW %
	Liaising	8.00	10.95	6.34	2.34	27.64
ACTIVITY	Planning	10.65	11.55	6.42	2.49	31.11
TYPES	Implementing	3.11	4.94	6.73	3.28	18.04
	Leading	3.37	2.24	12.08	5.52	23.21
	TOTAL COLUMN %	25.12	29.67	31.57	13.64	100%

The table shows the relative occurrence of activity–motive combinations. For example, the group of general managers see 'liaising' and 'planning' as activities which are primarily concerned with facilitating others' tasks and to a lesser extent their own tasks. Although both these activity types are also seen as a means of enhancing managers' own roles, they are not seen as an important means of enhancing the role of others in the organization. In contrast 'leading' is seen by the managers as being primarily functional in enhancing their own role although both task facilitation motives (i.e. own and others) are seen as relatively less important. 'Implementing' is characterized by a more balanced spread of motive types.

General managers differ not only on the activities they prefer to engage in but also with respect to the pattern of intentions which they consider is associated with different managerial activities.

Individual differences and an activity-motive for managers

The group data shown is based on all of the individual general managers' responses to the MAQ and as such 'masks' many of the individual differences in general managers' activity–motive patterns. In order to investigate the differences between general managers in greater detail each general manager's MAQ results were analyzed with respect to the 16 activity type/motive type combinations (as with the group results) and their weighted percentage scores determined for the 16 activity type/motive type combinations.

Based on their activity–motive preferences the managers in the sample fell into several distinct types, and it was apparent that some types of general manager are more inclined to pursue different sorts of organizational changes than managers of different activity–motive types. Notably, those general managers who predominantly preferred leading or planning activities to facilitate or enhance their own task performance were much more likely to pursue 'symbolic' rather than 'substantive' organizational changes. Symbolic changes are those which are primarily concerned with engendering awareness and acceptance of the new general management attitudes, ethos and culture. In contrast, those general managers who predominantly preferred liasing activities to facilitate their own task performance were more likely to pursue 'substantive' rather than symbolic organizational changes. Substantive changes are those which are primarily concerned with assessing and restructuring provisions and services.

Measure your activity-motive style

We have seen that there is an extremely wide range of activity–motive combinations which form part of the way in which general managers think about their jobs. By comparing and contrasting these activity–motive 'units' of managers' behaviour systems we have seen that there are a number of underlying general manager 'styles' and that managers with different styles tend to initiate different sorts of organizational change. These activity–motive styles are interesting since they may be related to other measures of managers' thinking styles and personality. As yet, these relationships have not been investigated, but we have developed a version of the MAQ which can provide an interesting focus for considering your own activity–motive style. The blank instrument, dubbed the MAMSC (Managers' Activity/Motive Style Checklist) is included and you may like to complete it. Instructions for scoring and interpretation are subsequently included using example data. The MAMSC may be used on an individual basis or the results may be combined for various sub-groups of managers in order to highlight different management approaches.

Manager's Activity/Motive Style Checklist (MAMSC)

How to complete the checklist

You will see below a list of 15 pairs of activities which briefly describe aspects of managerial work. You probably participate in most, if not all, of these activities in the course of your job. For the purposes of this exercise, assume if and where necessary that you participate in all of the activities listed below.

Each pair of activities is numbered 1 to 15 and members of each pair are distinguished by being labelled L (for left-hand activity) and R (for right-hand activity). You are asked to consider each pair of activities in turn and decide which one you prefer to engage in during the course of your job. Put a tick in either the left-hand box or the right-hand box of the answer sheet provided to show the activity you have chosen.

Following your choice of an activity within a pair, you are then required to give your reasons for choosing that particular activity. You will see on the answer sheet that there are 12 columns in the 'Reasons' section and these are labelled A to L. These 12 letters refer to the list of twelve reasons which are shown after the activity pairs below. For each of your chosen activities, tick those boxes which correspond to the reasons which support your choice of each activity pair. You must choose at least one reason for each choice but you may prefer to select several to support each of your preferences.

You must choose only one preferred activity from each pair. If you find it difficult to decide which activity you prefer, select the activity you spend more time engaged in.

There are no right or wrong answers and you are not being tested on your intelligence or ability. Remember to select only one activity of each pair and ensure that each of your activity choices is identified by the appropriate reasons.

ACTIVITY PAIRS

L (LEFT HAND)	ACTIVITY PAIR NUMBER	R (RIGHT HAND)
Maintaining your contact network	1	Expanding your contact network
Making decisions	2	Implementing decisions
Disseminating information	3	Receiving/monitoring information
Dealing with strategic organizational issues	4	Dealing with day-to-day organizational disturbances
Participating in unplanned informal face-to-face meetings	5	Participating in planned formal meetings

Engaging in long-range strategic planning	6	Engaging in short-range 'opportunistic' planning
Leading the organization	7	Acting as a spokesman/ figurehead for the organization
Controlling/directing subordinates	8	Briefing subordinates
Setting personal agendas for action	9	Controlling the organizational workflow
Dealing with general administrative duties	10	Dealing with matters requiring your specialist expertise
Allocating resources	11	Preserving assets
Initiating innovating activities	12	Participating in advisory or negotiating activities
Reviewing subordinates' progress	13	Setting your own job boundaries
Communicating with people at your level in the organization	14	Communicating with people not at your level in the organization
Asking/persuading people to do things	15	Telling/ordering people to do things

REASONS

(a) It helps me to achieve my own personal aims, objectives or goals.

(b) It facilitates others' enjoyment, interest or satisfaction.

(c) It enables others to fulfil the role expectations appropriately.

(d) It enhances my own enjoyment, interest or satisfaction.

(e) It enables others to be more effective or efficient.

(f) It enhances my own organizational understanding and influence.

(g) It helps others expand their impact or be more innovative.

(h) It enables me to be more effective or efficient.

(i) It helps others achieve their aims, objectives and goals.

(j) It enables me to fulfil the role expectations appropriately.

(k) It enhances others' organizational understanding and influence.

(l) It helps me expand my impact or be more innovative.

BLANK ANSWER SHEET

			REASONS FOR CHOOSING AN ACTIVITY											
LEFT HAND	PAIR NO.	RIGHT HAND	A	B	C	D	E	F	G	H	I	J	K	L
	1													
	2													
	3													
	4													
	5													
	6													
	7													
	8													
	9													
	10													
	11													
	12													
	13													
	14													
	15													

Scoring the checklist

The MAMSC is scored in two stages and an example of a completed
checklist is used in this section to demonstrate the scoring procedure.
Below is a completed answer sheet for a manager who had completed the
checklist (for the sake of clarity the manager's ticks have been replaced by
asterisks).

EXAMPLE MANAGER'S ANSWER SHEET

			REASONS FOR CHOOSING AN ACTIVITY											
LEFT HAND	PAIR NO.	RIGHT HAND	A	B	C	D	E	F	G	H	I	J	K	L
	1	★				★		★						★
★	2			★				★		★				
★	3				★		★					★		
★	4			★	★					★				★
★	5			★		★							★	
★	6			★			★	★				★		★
★	7			★		★		★				★		★
	8	★			★	★	★		★	★	★			★
★	9			★			★		★					★
	10	★				★				★		★		
★	11						★	★				★		★
★	12			★	★	★	★							★
	13	★	★			★				★		★		★
	14	★			★			★					★	★
★	15		★	★			★				★			

Scoring the answer sheet

The scoring key shown allocates every possible combination of responses to one of the 16 lower-case letters 'a' to 'p'. The first letter in each cell refers to the left-hand choice for any activity pair. The second letter in each cell refers to the right-hand choice for any activity pair. Each activity–reason combination selected is associated with a lower-case letter which is circled on the scoring key.

SCORING KEY

CHOICE PAIR	REASONS FOR CHOOSING AN ACTIVITY											
	A	B	C	D	E	F	G	H	I	J	K	L
1) L R	a/e	d/h	d/h	c/g	b/f	c/g	b/f	a/e	b/f	c/g	d/h	a/e
2) L R	m/i	p/l	p/l	o/k	n/j	o/k	n/j	m/i	n/j	o/k	p/l	m/i
3) L R	a/e	d/h	d/h	c/g	b/f	c/g	b/f	a/e	b/f	c/g	d/h	a/h
4) L R	m/i	p/l	p/l	o/k	n/j	o/k	n/j	m/i	n/j	o/k	p/1	m/i
5) L R	a/e	d/h	d/h	c/g	b/f	c/g	b/f	a/e	b/f	c/g	h/d	a/e
6) L R	e/e	h/h	h/h	g/g	f/f	g/g	f/f	e/e	f/f	g/g	h/h	e/e
7) L R	m/m	p/p	p/p	o/o	n/n	o/o	n/n	m/m	n/n	o/o	p/p	m/m
8) L R	i/i	l/l	l/l	k/k	j/j	k/k	j/j	i/i	j/j	k/k	l/l	i/i
9) L R	e/i	h/l	h/l	g/k	f/j	g/k	f/j	e/i	f/j	g/k	h/l	e/i
10) L R	i/m	l/p	l/p	k/o	j/n	k/o	j/n	i/m	j/n	k/o	l/p	i/m
11) L R	e/m	h/p	h/p	g/o	f/n	g/o	f/n	e/m	f/n	g/o	h/p	e/m
12) L R	i/a	l/d	l/d	k/c	j/b	k/c	j/b	i/a	j/b	k/c	l/d	i/a
13) L R	a/e	d/h	d/h	c/g	b/f	c/g	b/f	a/e	b/f	c/g	d/h	a/e
14) L R	a/a	d/d	d/d	c/c	b/b	c/c	b/b	a/a	b/b	c/c	d/d	a/a
15) L R	a/m	d/p	d/p	c/o	b/n	c/o	b/n	a/m	b/n	c/o	d/p	a/m

The next step is simply to count the frequency of each of the 16 circled letters. Since the liaising and planning activity types are each based on 8 MAMSC activities and the implementing and planning activities are each based on 7 MAMSC activities, it is necessary to weight the raw frequencies shown above by multiplying a–h by 7 and multiplying i–p by 8. These weighted frequencies are shown in brackets in table 9.4.

The next step is to convert each of the 6 weighted frequencies to a percentage of the grand total of weighted frequencies. This is shown in table 9.5, together with the marginal percentage totals. This weighted percentage table gives the activity–motive profile for our example manager with different managerial activity types being differentially associated with a different pattern of motives. The table summarizes the relative contribution of each of the four motive types for each of the activities which he has selected.

Table 9.4 Raw and weighted frequencies for each of the sixteen activity type/motive type categories for the example manager

		MOTIVE TYPES						
		FACILITATING				ENHANCING		
		Own tasks		Others' tasks		Own role		Others' role
ACTIVITY TYPES	Liaising	a = 4	(28)	b = 3	(21)	c = 3	(21)	d = 5 (35)
	Planning	e = 10	(70)	f = 3	(21)	g = 8	(56)	h = 0 (0)
	Implementing	i = 4	(32)	j = 4	(32)	k = 1	(8)	l = 4 (32)
	Leading	m = 8	(64)	n = 0	(0)	o = 6	(48)	p = 1 (8)

Table 9.5 Weighted percentage scores for each of the sixteen activity type/motive type categories for the example manager

		MOTIVE TYPES				
		FACILITATING		ENHANCING		
		Own tasks	Others' tasks	Own role	Others' role	TOTAL ROW %
ACTIVITY TYPES	Liaising	5.88	4.41	4.41	7.35	22.06
	Planning	14.71	4.41	11.76	0.00	30.88
	Implementing	6.72	6.72	1.68	6.72	21.83
	Leading	13.45	0.00	10.08	1.68	25.21
	TOTAL COLUMN %	40.76	15.55	27.94	15.76	100%

Interpreting the scores

We can see from the weighted percentage table that this manager's highest scores are for self-oriented items and in particular he views the activities of planning and leading as being useful in facilitating both his own task performance and enhancing his own organizational role. Interestingly, the activity-motive combination of leading to facilitate others' task performance was never selected by this manager. The combination leading to enhance others' organizational roles was also infrequently selected. Clearly this manager does not believe that leadership is particularly effective in changing others' roles or task performance. The activities of liaising and implementing are not particularly associated with any peaks or troughs in combination with the motive types, although liaising did occur relatively more frequently in conjunction with enhancing others' role in the organization, suggesting that the manager considered liaison as a moderately useful means of role enhancement for others.

When interpreting your own or others' scores you should examine and interpret the peaks and troughs in the profile as a means of focusing upon activity–motive style. However, it is worth remembering that any results should be treated with caution since this will remain an essentially intuitive process until adequate norms for the MAMSC are developed.

Concluding remarks

The results have demonstrated that what general managers do is related to what they expect to achieve. Further, the simultaneous analysis of managerial activities and motives can be used as a basis to develop a typology across all management contexts. This typology is broadly predictive of the actual programmes of organizational changes which general managers are planning or implementing in their own districts and units, although it must be remembered that all individual general managers possess a unique set of perceptions in guiding their organizational behaviour.

The proposed typology is in its infancy and currently merely reflects general managers' relative emphasis on different activity–motive combinations. Much work remains to be undertaken but dealing with activity–motive combinations as the 'unit' of managerial work may have a great deal of potential, particularly in furthering our understanding of what exactly constitutes 'effective' general management. As Hales (1986) has observed, the problem of much of the managerial research to date has been the reluctance to ask why managers behave in the way they do. Understanding the conceptual frameworks which underpin managerial activities could have important implications for assessing the performance of general managers. The key to understanding managerial effectiveness may lie within the 'appropriateness' of the correspondence between what managers actually do and why they choose to behave in that way.

CHAPTER 10

The path to managing change

Throughout this text we have tried to illustrate the integrated nature of general management and the management of change. In particular the early chapters were concerned with understanding the background to the Griffiths Inquiry and then to the nature of general management itself (Chapters 1, 2 and 3). This was followed we hope logically, by an exploration of the theoretical approaches to the process of organizational change (Chapter 4). In this chapter it was evident that despite our attempts to impose a classificatory structure upon the various approaches they remain complex, overlapping and potentially confusing. It is not easy to see what practical steps a manager should take after assimilating these various options. Indeed, we would argue that the conceptual and theoretical separation of models of management from models of change is a major contributor to this state of affairs.

In recent years the literature and provision of courses directed towards the management of change have proliferated. Managers, quite rightly recognizing the key role of organizational change, have been keen to seek solutions from the diversity of advice and support offered. However, we believe that attempting to separate the management of change from 'normal' management is fundamentally flawed thinking. Managers are managing change all the time. Organizations are never static whether one is concerned with physical or human resources or reshaping the organizational focus by responding to a constantly changing external environment. This view is reinforced when we consider the nature of day-to-day general management – fragmented, superficial, dealing with a whole range of issues. Whether coping with everyday operational issues or developing a strategic vision of a new organization, a manager is continuously managing change – small or large scale, short or long term. The need therefore is to provide an integrative structure whereby management and change management can be seen as unified processes. We believe understanding the individual manager's mental models as described here provides an important means for achieving this integration. Before examining the uses of this approach in more detail it is important to recognize the increasing pressures within the NHS to be able to handle far-reaching, rapid change as well as maintaining the current level of service provision. The problems of integrating maintenance and change management are becoming increasingly apparent.

New pressures for integrated change management

The publication of the government's White Paper 'Working for Patients' (1989) is as clear an index of the pressures for change as one could imagine. There may be some debate as to whether the ideas set out in these documents are again part of an evolving philosophy of central government's view of the Health Service or whether they are new ideas discontinuous with the past. As ever there is surely an element of both but what cannot be disputed is that the degree of change implied is profound. The proposals suggest radical changes in the way the NHS is funded and in some instances dramatically alter the type of organization the managers are expected to manage. Both consultants within hospitals and general practitioners in the community are likely to be deeply affected by the new structures. It is, of course, by no means certain that the White Paper will be implemented in its proposed form. The BMA has consistently rejected the government's plans and is in the midst of a high profile national campaign against the implementation of the White Paper. Similarly the professional representative body of the general practitioners has voted to reject the new conditions of service. The prospect now exists of these contracts being imposed in a 'take it or leave it' style.

It is not the intention here to review the host of commentaries, criticisms, support and questions that have emerged following the publication of the White Paper. Rather one or two examples of the implied changes will be cited to illustrate the sort of change the NHS may have to embrace.

One clear and fundamental change is the separation of the supply role in health care from that of demand or commission. Thus District Health Authorities may radically alter their stance to become commissioning agents on behalf of the population they serve. They would seek to contract for the type of services needed by this population on the most favourable quality and cost terms available. The providers of such services are likely to be many of the units that once formed part of the District Authority itself together with direct provision from any other suitable public or private source. Some of these units may acquire what the White Paper describes as self-governing hospital status whilst others will remain as part of the District itself. This proposed arrangement results in many queries and ambiguities about the relationships as yet unanswered by the government. For example, in those Districts where units remain part of the District structure it appears quite possible for a District General Manager to simultaneously have a clear and rigorously defined contract for services (with explicit penalty clauses presumably) as well as having a line management relationship with the Unit General Manager of a particular unit. What happens if a key general hospital in an isolated geographic position fails to deliver on the specified contract? Does it lose money through withdrawal of contracts until it is no longer viable and is forced to close? This would seem to be the logical impact of market forces, but if patients now have to travel twice as far to receive treatment it is difficult to see how patient choice has been improved.

Whatever the detailed outcome of the proposals in practice it is clear from this one example that vast organizational changes are set in motion. In summary we could posit the following changes in structure and skills required that managers will need to consider.

District Commissioning Authorities

Must create the skills to:

a) Identify relatively and precisely the demands of its population served. Unfortunately the quality of this type of population data is probably incapable of anything less than generalized statement;
b) Specify tight, enforceable contracts with providers to meet these needs. Not only is the data from (a) limited but so too are the existing skills in service contracting;
c) Monitor and regulate any such contracts in terms of cost and quality of service provided. This too becomes problematic when one considers the range of factors that may need to be taken into account. The private sector has for many years invested a great deal in highly trained staff and sophisticated techniques to monitor its purchasing agreements. Will such staff exist in a slimmed-down District Health Authority?
d) Liaise closely with Family Practitioner Committees and the general practitioners who will become the front line in defining the needs of the population and in utilizing the service contracts agreed by the Districts.

There are many other changes of course, notably the likely reduction of provider services at District level. Changes though in the nature of the organization are considerable as are the new skills that now become critical.

At unit level, too, similar repercussions can be seen. Clearly units must now place great emphasis upon marketing the services they wish to sell. Consequently, they must know how to price these services accurately and realistically and they must develop the ability to measure the quality of their service at any level and in any sphere demanded by the customer.

Again the level of change is obvious and serves to highlight the emphasis given in the White Paper to the local structure. It is possible in this scenario for managers at a local level to develop the structures and systems to supply the service they define. This is, of course, an exciting challenge. It also perhaps provides an impetus to greater diversity, fragmentation and possible future break-up of the NHS.

A further example of change implied in the White Paper is the emphasis given to medical audit which has become almost indistiguishably intertwined with resource management

Within hospitals in particular, consultants are being encouraged to carefully examine their practices and to consider their appropriateness along a whole range of quality measures from process factors to outcome. Many clinicians have of course undertaken such a procedure either individually or with colleagues for some time. Many welcome the impetus given to this type of monitoring. However, others are less comfortable with an almost unavoidable link between measures of medical activity and the associated costs. In order to involve clinicians in management such a process is essential. Clinicians are the allocators of resources and it is entirely legitimate to ask that they understand how the decisions they make affect the use of scarce resources.

As information about medical practice becomes more precise it is easier to see just how money is being spent, and it is also legitimate to ask whether some savings could be made. However, and this is where the tension exists for clinicians, is it legitimate to ask clinicians to consider the cost element if there is any likelihood that it may reduce the quality of care given to patients. We see here the uneasy interface between managers and clinicians reflected in whether the emphasis upon quality of care and efficiency in delivery of care are compatible. The attraction of resource management is that it offers the service a systematic way of establishing the basis of its costs and with the increased likelihood of competition between hospitals it will be virtually impossible to resist.

Once again significant change can be seen in the whole fabric of organizational dynamics with the emergence of clinical directors to co-ordinate and manage groupings of clinical activity at a very senior level of management. The future interaction between powerful and effective clinical directors and unit general managers will be observed with interest.

A similar restructuring of activities will occur with general practitioners whether they hold practice budgets or not. The tension between cost and quality of care remains unresolved. One of the great unknowns is how the relationship between primary and secondary care will be handled. Just how will the new and strengthened FHSA's interact with District Health Authorities? Is there really a case for merging the two bodies around more clearly defined geographical and population parameters?

A wide range of issues could be explored here, such as the role and function of non-executive directors on health authorities. However, the point to be made is that change is just part of management and the volume of change at present is tremendous.

Using this book to tackle change

Our aim in preparing this book has been to help managers understand the factors that influence them as general managers and as those directly responsible for initiating and shaping how their organization responds to internal and external pressures.

We have stated that we do not believe an adequate prescriptive model of change exists. Both the wide-ranging nature of organizations and the individual goals and expectations of change agents make such prescriptive, procedural approaches to creating change unrealistic. Understanding organizational change is more a question of attempting to make the internal mental models of change agents explicit and examining how the organization is seen at present and how it is expected to develop in the future. This process is represented in the diagrammatic model presented in Figure 10.1. A brief expansion of the stages of the model will make explicit how each of the chapters in the book seeks to help in the various phases.

We have argued that it is not enough to understand what managers do. We also need to know how the manager views the change process and the goals, values and expectations upon which this process is founded. The key to this is an effective Stage 1 where managers seek to establish an accurate and clear picture of what the organization is like at present (Items (a), (b) and (c) of Stage 1) and integrate this with the vision in Item (d). Many standard techniques exist for compiling information about (a), (b) and (c), but assessing (d) is a more difficult issue. Some would argue that this 'vision' is intuitive and is a form of mental functioning only available to some managers. This ability to create a vision of the future organization may be an important distinguishing feature of the outstanding manager. Specifically, this ability may prove to be the key aspect of leadership in management whilst ensuring the spread and understanding of what this vision means to all employees may imply a range of other attributes.

Following through to Stage II of the model we can see that this stage is dominated by the internal representation of events. From established facts and ideas the manager maintains a monitoring role which has a strong selective attention aspect in which key problem areas are defined, scanned or examined. Implicitly, the vision of change directs the monitoring behaviour and is made compatible with the desired change outcomes by an increasing awareness of the strategy and a mental rehearsal of what needs to be done. Stage II, Formulation, is characterized by the cognitive effort to minimize incompatibility between the vision of change and the desired outcomes of a change strategy. The instruments in Chapters 6 and 7 are geared to help managers interrogate their own thinking in this crucial area.

Stage III is about implementation and is where the mental model is transformed into declared goals, and specific outcomes. There is a tremendous load upon communication at this stage because much of the analysis has been accomplished. There are also key practical skills and knowledge about procedures and systems that can be critical to effectiveness in this Stage. Obviously there must always be a monitoring of feedback aspect to this final element so that deviations from the model can be examined and incorporated where appropriate.

Aspects of the theories of change discussed in Chapter 4 may be useful in describing this entire process but it is the individual manager's mental model which determines the strategy of how the elements of these stages are tackled. Consistent and compatible movement towards the desired change is the hallmark of the effective manager. Managers involved in change, at all levels of the organization, might benefit by examining how they are proceeding through this process. The guides in Chapters 6 and 7 will help in this diagnosis, as might the research in Chapters 8 and 9 which outlines how others have fared. It is clear from this research that the consequence of inadequate mental models can seriously constrain the effectiveness of planned programmes of change. Only by an integration of mental models with change initiatives will the organization move forward effectively.

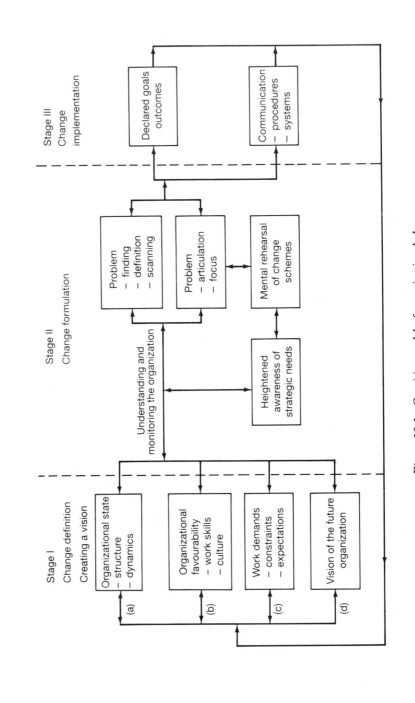

Figure 10.1 Cognitive model of organizational change

Appendix – Copy of measures used in the investigation

Perception of organizational change

Instructions

The Scale consists of eighteen items relating to general features of organizational change. Each of the eighteen items has two parts.

1   The first part relates to that part of the organization for which you personally have responsibility. This is referred to as 'your part of the organization' in the rating scale.
2. The second part of the item relates to the organization as a whole.

Please rate parts (1) and (2) for each of the following conditions

  (a) **Present**   –   How you perceive your organization to be at the present time
  (b) **Future**   –   How you think your organization is likely to be in three years' time
  (c) **Preferred** –   How you would prefer your organization to be in three years' time.

There are no right or wrong answers. When completing each part of an item in the rating scale carefully place a cross (X) anywhere along each 'rating line' at the point which best represents where your opinion lies for each of the three conditions. The ends of each 'rating line' represent the point at which only one end of a dimension applies. The centre position of each 'rating line' represents the point at which both ends of the dimension apply equally.

Please try to rate parts (1.) and (2.) of all eighteen items on the three conditions. However, if you really cannot complete a particular item please rate as not applicable.

Perception of organizational change scale

Please rate the following.

1. (a) Rate the degree to which your part of the organization has the

capacity to respond to changes induced directly or indirectly by other parts of the organization.

		Extremely unresponsive			Extremely responsive
(A)	PRESENT	I_____I
(B)	FUTURE	I_____I
(C)	PREFERRED	I_____I

1. (b) Rate the degree to which your organization as a whole has the capacity to respond to changes induced by the environment external to the organization.

		Extremely unresponsive			Extremely responsive
(A)	PRESENT	I_____I
(B)	FUTURE	I_____I
(C)	PREFERRED	I_____I

2. (a) Rate the extent to which your own management activities utilize setting objectives and planning as methods of controlling your part of the organization.

		Not at all reliant			Extremely reliant
(A)	PRESENT	I_____I
(B)	FUTURE	I_____I
(C)	PREFERRED	I_____I

2. (b) Rate the extent to which you consider management as a whole utilizes setting objectives and planning as methods of controlling the organization.

		Not at all reliant			Extremely reliant
(A)	PRESENT	I_____I
(B)	FUTURE	I_____I
(C)	PREFERRED	I_____I

3. (a) Rate the degree to which the internal structures of your part of the organization are fixed and permanent.

		Rigid/unchanging structure		Temporary changeable structure
(A)	PRESENT	I_____I		
(B)	FUTURE	I_____I		
(C)	PREFERRED	I_____I		

3. (b) Rate the degree to which the internal structures of the organization as a whole are fixed and permanent.

		Rigid/unchanging structure		Temporary/ changeable structure
(A)	PRESENT	I_____I		
(B)	FUTURE	I_____I		
(C)	PREFERRED	I_____I		

4. (a) Rate the extent to which your own management activities utilize written policies and procedures as methods of controlling your part of the organization.

		Extremely reliant		Not at all reliant
(A)	PRESENT	I_____I		
(B)	FUTURE	I_____I		
(C)	PREFERRED	I_____I		

4. (b) Rate the extent to which management as a whole utilizes written policies and procedures as methods of organization control.

		Extremely reliant		Not at all reliant
(A)	PRESENT	I_____I		
(B)	FUTURE	I_____I		
(C)	PREFERRED	I_____I		

5. (a) Within your part of the organization, to what extent can significant organizational change be identified and assessed?

		Not at all		Very well
(A)	PRESENT	I_____		I
(B)	FUTURE	I_____		I
(C)	PREFERRED	I_____		I

5. (b) To what extent can the significant organizational change be identified and assessed within the organization as a whole?

		Not at all	Very well
(A)	PRESENT	I_____I	
(B)	FUTURE	I_____I	
(C)	PREFERRED	I_____I	

6. (a) Rate the extent to which your own managerial problem-solving utilizes past experience of similar problems or focuses on the current emerging needs of your part of the organization.

		Totally based on past experience	Totally based on emerging needs
(A)	PRESENT	I_____I	
(B)	FUTURE	I_____I	
(C)	PREFERRED	I_____I	

6. (b) In general, rate the extent to which you feel problem-solving by management as a whole utilizes past experience of similar problems or focuses on the current emerging needs of the organization as a whole.

		Totally based on past experience	Totally based on emerging needs
(A)	PRESENT	I_____I	
(B)	FUTURE	I_____I	
(C)	PREFERRED	I_____I	

7. (a) In general, rate the manner in which you react to proposed change to that part of the organization for which you are responsible.

		Always accept and facilitate proposed change	Always reject and block proposed change
(A)	PRESENT	I_____I	
(B)	FUTURE	I_____I	
(C)	PREFERRED	I_____I	

7. (b) Rate the manner in which you feel management as a whole reacts to proposed organizational change.

		Always accepts and facilitates proposed change	Always rejects and blocks proposed change
(A)	PRESENT	I_____I	
(B)	FUTURE	I_____I	
(C)	PREFERRED	I_____I	

8. (a) In general, within your part of the organization, rate the extent to which you consider that the power effectively to implement organizational change rests with the formal power holders or with other informal power holders.

		Power totally informal	Power totally formal
(A)	PRESENT	I_____	_____I
(B)	FUTURE	I_____	_____I
(C)	PREFERRED	I_____	_____I

8. (b) Within the organization as a whole rate the extent to which you consider that the power effectively to implement organization change rests with the formal power holders or with other informal power holders.

		Power totally informal	Power totally formal
(A)	PRESENT	I_____	_____I
(B)	FUTURE	I_____	_____I
(C)	PREFERRED	I_____	_____I

9. (a) How frequently do changes occurring in other parts of the organization affect the stability of that part of the organization for which you are responsible?

		Extremely frequently	Extremely infrequently
(A)	PRESENT	I_____	_____I
(B)	FUTURE	I_____	_____I
(C)	PREFERRED	I_____	_____I

9. (b) How frequently do changes in the wider external environment affect the stability of your organization as a whole?

		Extremely frequently	Extremely infrequently
(A)	PRESENT	I_____	_____I
(B)	FUTURE	I_____	_____I
(C)	PREFERRED	I_____	_____I

10. (a) In your part of the organization rate the extent to which you consider that the internal organizational structure has been planned or allowed to evolve.

		Completely planned	Completely evolved
(A)	PRESENT	I_____	I
(B)	FUTURE	I_____	I
(C)	PREFERRED	I_____	I

10. (b) For the organization as a whole, rate the extent to which you consider that the internal organizational structure has been planned or allowed to evolve.

		Completely planned	Completely evolved
(A)	PRESENT	I_____	I
(B)	FUTURE	I_____	I
(C)	PREFERRED	I_____	I

11. (a) Rate the extent to which your own management activities utilize systems of financial monitoring as methods of controlling your part of the organization.

		Not at all reliant	Extremely reliant
(A)	PRESENT	I_____	I
(B)	FUTURE	I_____	I
(C)	PREFERRED	I_____	I

11. (b) Rate the extent to which you consider management as a whole utilizes systems of financial monitoring as methods of controlling the organization.

		Not at all reliant	Extremely reliant
(A)	PRESENT	I_____	I
(B)	FUTURE	I_____	I
(C)	PREFERRED	I_____	I

12. (a) In your part of the organization rate the extent to which you attempt to implement novel solutions to organizational problems which have not been tried before.

		All novel solutions		All previously tried solutions
(A)	PRESENT	I		I
(B)	FUTURE	I		I
(C)	PREFERRED	I		I

12. (b) Rate the extent to which you consider management as a whole attempts to implement novel solutions to organizational problems which have not been tried before.

		All novel solutions		All previously tried solutions
(A)	PRESENT	I		I
(B)	FUTURE	I		I
(C)	PREFERRED	I		I

13. (a) Rate the extent to which the standards against which the performance of your part of the organization is measured reflect traditional stable criteria or novel innovatory criteria.

		Traditional stable criteria		Novel innovatory criteria
(A)	PRESENT	I		I
(B)	FUTURE	I		I
(C)	PREFERRED	I		I

13. (b) In general, rate the extent to which the standards against which the performance of the organization as a whole is measured reflect traditional stable criteria or novel innovatory criteria.

		Traditional stable criteria		Novel innovatory criteria
(A)	PRESENT	I		I
(B)	FUTURE	I		I
(C)	PREFERRED	I		I

14. (a) Generally, within your part of the organization do you consider that important communication travels through formal or informal channels?

		Completely informal channels	Completely formal channels
(A)	PRESENT	I_____I	
(B)	FUTURE	I_____I	
(C)	PREFERRED	I_____I	

14. (b) Within the organization as a whole, do you consider that important communication travels through formal or informal channels?.

		Completely informal channels	Completely formal channels
(A)	PRESENT	I_____I	
(B)	FUTURE	I_____I	
(C)	PREFERRED	I_____I	

15. (a) Rate the extent to which your efforts are directed towards issues internal to or external to that part of the organization for which you are responsible.

		Effort totally internal	Effort totally external
(A)	PRESENT	I_____I	
(B)	FUTURE	I_____I	
(C)	PREFERRED	I_____I	

15. (b) Rate the extent to which management as a whole generally directs its efforts toward issues internal or external to the organization as a whole.

		Effort totally internal	Effort totally external
(A)	PRESENT	I_____I	
(B)	FUTURE	I_____I	
(C)	PREFERRED	I_____I	

16. (a) Within your part of the organization, rate the extent to which you consider that individuals have the freedom to structure their own jobs.

		Great deal of individual freedom	No individual freedom
(A)	PRESENT	I_____I	
(B)	FUTURE	I_____I	
(C)	PREFERRED	I_____I	

16. (b) Within the organization as a whole, rate the extent to which you consider that individuals have the freedom to structure their own jobs.

		Great deal of individual freedom	No individual freedom
(A)	PRESENT	I_____	I
(B)	FUTURE	I_____	I
(C)	PREFERRED	I_____	I

17. (a) Rate the extent to which your part of the organization is able to predict and anticipate significant future changes in the organization as a whole.

		Not able at all	Extremely able
(A)	PRESENT	I_____	I
(B)	FUTURE	I_____	I
(C)	PREFERRED	I_____	I

17. (b) To what extent do you consider the organization as a whole is able to predict and anticipate significant future changes in the wider external environment?

		Not able at all	Extremely able
(A)	PRESENT	I_____	I
(B)	FUTURE	I_____	I
(C)	PREFERRED	I_____	I

18. (a) When organizational change is introduced into your part of the organization, to what extent do you consider that it is important to ensure continuity with past organization structures and procedures?

		Not at all important	Extremely important
(A)	PRESENT	I_____	I
(B)	FUTURE	I_____	I
(C)	PREFERRED	I_____	I

18. (b) In general, when organization change is introduced, to what extent do you consider that management as a whole feels it is important to ensure continuity with past organizational structures and procedures?

		Not at all important	Extremely important
(A)	PRESENT	I_____	I
(B)	FUTURE	I_____	I
(C)	PREFERRED	I_____	I

****

THANK YOU FOR YOUR CO-OPERATION

Please complete Section II

Section II

Instructions for completing the list of key changes table

The rating scale you have just completed is concerned with a range of factors relating to organizational change in general terms. In order to provide some context for your ratings, the second part of this exercise requires you to list some specific critical changes which are or will be taking place in your organization in the foreseeable future.

In the list of Key Changes Table you are requested to briefly list as few or as many changes that you feel important, describing each one with not more that a sentence or two of your own words. There is enough space to include six changes in all and this is the maximum number you are asked to describe. NB If you feel only one or two changes are relevant do not attempt to complete six.

After you have briefly described a key change, rate the change you have described with respect to the three dimensions shown. These dimensions relate to

(a) The speed at which you feel each change is or will be occurring.
(b) The degree of personal involvement you have or will have in implementing the change.
(c) The degree of personal commitment you have towards each change.

You rate each change as before, by carefully placing a cross on the 'rating line' at the point at which you consider best describes where each of your listed changes lie.

Section III

Managerial activities questionnaire

Below is a list of 15 pairs of activities which briefly describe aspects of managerial work. You probably participate in most, if not all, of these activities in the course of your job. For the purposes of this exercise, assume if and where necessary that you participate in all the activities listed below.

Look at each pair of activities and decide which you prefer to do and put a tick in either the left-hand box or the right-hand box on the answer sheet provided to show the activity you have chosen.

Then give your reasons for choosing that activity or rejecting the other one.

If you are unable to decide which activity you prefer, do not tick either box, but explain why you either like or dislike both of them.

There are no right or wrong answers, but try to avoid vague answers such as 'interesting', 'satisfying', 'boring', 'I like it', 'I prefer it', etc.

Please proceed now to check each statement plus supplying your reasons.

L (LEFT HAND)	ACTIVITY PAIR NUMBER	R (RIGHT HAND)
Maintaining your contact network	1	Expanding your contact network
Making decisions	2	Implementing decisions
Disseminating information	3	Receiving/monitoring information
Dealing with strategic organizational issues	4	Dealing with day-to-day organizational disturbances
Participating in unplanned informal face-to-face meetings	5	Participating in planned formal meetings
Engaging in long-range strategic planning	6	Engaging in short-range 'opportunistic' planning
Leading the organization	7	Acting as a spokesman/figurehead for the organization
Controlling/directing subordinates	8	Briefing subordinates
Setting personal agendas for action	9	Controlling the organizational workflow
Dealing with general administrative duties	10	Dealing with matters requiring your specialist expertise
Allocating resources	11	Preserving assets
Initiating innovating activities	12	Participating in advisory or negotiating activities
Reviewing subordinates' progress	13	Setting your own job boundaries
Communicating with people at your level in the organization	14	Communicating with people not at your level in the organization
Asking/persuading people to do things	15	Telling/ordering people to do things

Answer sheet

Managerial activities questionnaire

NAME .... ORGANIZATION ....

DATE .... SEX /M/F ....

JOB TITLE .... AGE ....

Left hand	Pair no.	Right hand	Reason for choosing or rejecting
	1		
	2		
	3		
	4		
	5		
	6		
	7		
	8		
	9		
	10		
	11		
	12		
	13		
	14		
	15		

References

Abel-Smith B. (1976). *Value for Money in Health Services*. London, Heinemann.

Ackoff R.L. (1967). Management misinformation systems. *Management Science* December: 147–56.

Aguilar F.J. (1988). *General Managers in Action*. New York, Oxford University Press.

Allen D. and Lupton T. (1988). Contingency theory, the introduction of general management into the health service. *Management Education and Development* 14: Part I: 47–50.

Alleyway L. (1987) Beating a hasty retreat. *Nursing Times*; 83(36): 18–20.

Andrews K.R. (1980). *The Concept of Corporate Strategy*. Homewood, R.D. Irwin, US.

Argyris C. and Schon D.A. (1978). *Organisation Learning: A Theory of Action Perspective*. Reading, Mass., Addison Wesley.

Axelrod R.(1976). *The Structure of Decisions: Cognitive Maps of Political Elites*. Princeton, NJ, Princeton University Press.

Beckhard R. (1969) *Organisational Development: Strategies and Models*, Reading, Mass., Addison Wesley.

Beckhard R. (1985). *Managing Change in Organisations: Participants' Workbook*. Reading, Mass., Addison Wesley.

Bell G. (1967). Formality vs. flexibility in complex organisations. In G. Bell (ed), *Organisations and Human Behaviour*. Englewood Cliffs, NJ, Prentice-Hall, pp. 97–106.

Bennis W. (1969). *Organisation Development: Its Nature, Origins and Prospects*. Reading, Mass., Addison Wesley.

Bergwerk J.M. and Clarke A. (1982). *The Job Feature Questionnaire Manual*. ITRU Ltd.

Best G. (1984). *General Management: An Audit for Commitment and Action*. NHSTA Occasional Papers 1. Godalming, Surrey, NHSTA.

Blake R.R. and Mouton J.S. (1968). *Corporate Excellence Through Grid Organisation Development*. Gulf Publishing.

Bourgon M.G. (1983). Uncovering cognitive maps: the self-q technique. In Morgan, G. (ed), *Beyond Method*. Beverly Hills, Calif., Sage.

Bowden D. (1988). Management, the Institute and the NHS. IHSM Presidential Address. *Health Service Management*; 84(4): 64–8.

Braybrooke D. and Lindbolm C.E. (1963). *A Strategy of Decision*. New York, Free Press.

Brewer E. and Tomlinson, J.W.C. (1964). The manager's working day. *Journal of Industrial Economics*; 12: 191–7.

Brill P. and Pierskalla C. (1982). Issues in the application of organisation development in health care organisatins. In Margulies and Adams (eds), *Organisation Development in Health Organisations*. Reading, Mass., Addison Wesley.

Burgoyne J. and Stuart R. (1976). The nature, use and acquisition of managerial skills and other attributes. *Personnel Review*; 5(4): 19–29.

Burns T. and Stalker G.M. (1961). *The Management of Innovation*. London, Tavistock.

Chandler A.D. (1962). *Strategy and Structure*. Cambridge, Mass., MIT Press.

Clegg C.W. (1982). Modelling the practice of job redesign. In J.E. Kelly and C.W. Clegg (eds), *Autonomy and Control at the Workplace: Contexts for Job Redesign*. London, Croom Helm.

Clifton-Williams J. (1978). *Human Behaviour in Organisations*. South Western Publishing Co.

Cohen M.D. and March J.G. (1974). *Leadership and Ambiguity: The American College President*. New York, McGraw-Hill.

Cohen M.D., March J.G. and Olsen, J.P. (1976). People, problems, solutions and the ambiguity of relevance. In J.G. March and J.P. Owen, *Ambiguity and Choice in Organisations*. Bergen, Universiteit Sforlaget.

Crozier M. (1964). *The Bureaucratic Phenomenon*. London, Tavistock Publishing Co.

Cyert R.L. and March J.G. (1963). *A Behavioural Theory of the Firm*. Englewood Cliffs, Prentice Hall.

Dalton M. (1959). *Men who Manage*. New York, Wiley.

Dearden J. (1972). MIS is a mirage. *Harvard Business Review*; 50(1): 90–99.

Dimmock S. (1985). The role of the general manager. *Nursing Times*; February 6.

Disken S., Dixon M. and Halpern S. (1987). The new UGMs – an analysis of management at unit level. *The Health Service Journal*; July, 1–8.

Downs G.W.R. Jnr and Mohr L.B. (1976). Conceptual issues in the study of innovation. *Administrative Science Quarterly*; 21.

Duncan R. (1973). Multiple decision making structures in adapting to environmental uncertainty: the impact on organisational effectiveness. *Human Relations*; 26: 273–92.

Dutton J., Fahey L. and Narayanan V. (1983). Toward understanding strategic issue diagnosis. *Strategic Management Journal*; 4: 307–23.

Edmonstone J. (1985). The values problem in O.D. *Leadership and Organisational Department Journal*, 6: 2.

Egan G. (1985). *Change Agent Skills in Helping and Human Service Settings*. Brooks/Cole.

Etzioni A. (1973). Mixed scanning: a third approach to decision making. In A. Falude (ed), *A Reader in Planning Theory*. Oxford, Pergamon Press. (First published in *Public Administration Domain*; December 1967.)

Feldman S.P. (1986). Management in context: an essay on the relevance of culture to the understanding of organisational change. *Journal of Management Studies*; 23: 6 November.

Ferlie E. and McKee L. (1988). *Planning for alternative futures in the NHS* Health Services Research Management (1): March, 4–18.

Fitter M.J. (1982). Information systems and the organisational implications of job redesign. In J.E. Kelly and C.W. Clegg (eds), *Autonomy and Control of the Workplace: Contexts for Job Redesign*. London, Croom Helm, pp 129–56.

Flanagan H. and Spurgeon P. (1988). On being effective. *Hospital and Health Services Review*; April: 67–69.

French W.L. and Bell, C.H. (1973) *Organisation development: behavioural science interventions for organisation improvement*. Englewood Cliffs, Prentice Hall.

Friedlander F. (1976). O.D. reaches adolescence:. an exploration of underlying values. *Journal of Applied Behavioural Science*; 12(1): January–March.

Fry R.E. (1982). Improving trustee, administrator and physician collaboration through open systems planning. In Margulies and Adams (eds), *Organisational Development in Health Care Organisations*. Reading, Mass., Addison Wesley.

Gagliardi P. (1986). The creation and change of organisational cultures: a conceptual framework. *Organisation Studies*; 7(2): 117–34.

Galbraith J.R. (1974). Organisation design: an information processing view. *TIMS Interfaces*; 4(3): 28–36.

Gillem D.J. and Carroll S.J. (1985). Relationships of managerial ability to unit effectiveness in more organic versus more mechanistic departments. *Journal of Management Studies*; 22(6); 668–76.

Greiner L.E. (1967). Patterns of organisation change. *Harvard Business Review*; May–June: 119–28.

Greiner L.E. (1982). Senior executives as strategic actors. Paper presented at Research Seminar on Strategy, Helsinki School of Economics, Helsinki, Finland, June.

Grinyer P. and Norburn D. (1975). Planning for existing markets: perceptions of executives and financial performance. *Journal of the Royal Statistical Society*; 3(1): 47–64.

Gunn L. (1989). A public management approach to the NHS. *Health Services Management Research*; 2(1).

Hague E.J. and Aiken, N. (1970). *Social Change in Complex Organisations*. New York, Random House.

Hage J. (1980). *Theories of Organisations: Form, Process and Transformation*. New York, Wiley.

Hales C.P. (1986). What do managers do? A critical review of the evidence. *Journal of Management Studies*; 23(1): 88–115.

Hales C.P. (1987). The manager's work in context: a pilot investigation of the relationship between managerial role demands and role performance. *Personnel Review*; 16(5): 26–33.

Handy C.B. (1976). *Understanding Organisations*. Harmondsworth, Penguin.

Handy C. (1989). *The Age of Unreason*. London, Hutchinson.

Harman H.H. (1976). *Modern Factor Analysis*. Third Edition. University of Chicago Press.

Harrison M.I. (1987). *Diagnosing Organisations: Methods, Models and Processes*. Applied Social Research Methods Series, Vol. 8. Sage Publications Inc.

Harrison S. The workforce and the new managerialism, pp. 141–152; Parston G. Evolution – general management, pp. 17–33. In Maxwell R. (ed), (1988), *Reshaping the National Health Service*. Berkshire, Policy Journals.

Harrison S., Hunter D.J., Marnoch G. and Pollitt P., (1989). General management and medical autonomy in the National Health Service. *Health Services Management Research*; 2(1): 38–46.

Hartley J., Kelly J.E. and Nicholson N. (1983). *Steel Strike: A Case Study in Industrial Relations*. London, Batsford, Academic and Educational.

Hartley M.J. (1988). Performance indicators in the management process. *Health Services Management Research*; 1(1): 29–42.

Herbst P.G. (1970). *Behavioural worlds. The study of single cases*. London, Tavistock Publications.

Hickman C.R. and Silva, A. (1984). *Creating Excellence: Merging Corporate Culture, Strategy and Change in the New Age*. London, Allen & Unwin.

Hirsh W. and Bevan S. (1988). *What Makes a Manager?* Institute of Manpower Studies Report no. 144, Brighton, Sussex.

Hofstede E. (1986). Editorial: the usefulness of the 'organisational culture' concept. *Journal of Management Studies*; 23(3): 253–7.

Hogarth R.M. (1980). *Judgement and Choice: the Psychology of Decisions*. Chichester, Wiley.

Hopwood A. (1974). *Accounting and Human Behaviour*. London, Haymarket Publishing Ltd.

Horne J.H. and Lupton N.T. (1965). The work activities of middle managers: an exploratory study. *Journal of Management Studies*; 2(1); 14–33.

Hosking D.M. and Morley L.E. (1985). The skills of leadership. Paper presented to the Eighth Biennial Leadership Symposium, Texas Tech. University, Texas, USA. July 23–7.

Kable J.C. (1986). Decision perception analysis – measuring a manager's preference for managing. *Journal of Management Development*; 2(3); 3–18.

Kahn R.L. (1974). Organisation developments: some problems and proposals. *Journal of Applied Behavioural Science*; 10(4); 485–502.

Kanter R.M. (1983). *The Change Masters: Innovation for Productivity in the American Corporation*. New York, Simon E. Schuster.

Kast F.E. and Rosenweig, J.E. (1985). *Organisation and Management: A Systems and Contingency Approach*. New York, McGraw-Hill.

Kelly G.A. (1955). *The Psychology of Personal Constructs*. Vols 1 and 2. New York, Norton.

Kirton M.J. (1987). *Kirton Adaption-Innovation Inventory*. Hatfield, UK, Occupational Research Centre.

Klein R. (1985). Management in health care: the politics of innovation. *International Journal of Health Planning and Management*; 1: 57–63.

Kotter J. (1978). *Organisation dynamics*. Reading, Mass., Addison Wesley.

Kotter J.P. (1982) *The General Managers*. New York, Free Press.

Lawrence P.R. and Lorsch J.W. (1969). *Developing Organisations: Diagnosis and Action*. Reading, Mass., Addison Wesley.

Leavitt M.J. (1964). Applied organizational change in industry: structural, technical and human approaches. In W.W. Cooper, H.J. Leavitt and M.W. Shelly II (eds), *New Perspectives in Organisation Research*. New York, Wiley.

Legge K. (1984). *Evaluating Planned Organisational Change*. London, Academic Press.

Lindblom C.E. (1959). The science of muddling through. *Public Administration Review*; 10(2): 79–99.

Lutmans F., Rosenkratz S.A. and Hennessy M.W. (1985). What do successful managers really do? An observation study of managerial activities. *Institute of Applied Behaviour Science*; 21(3): 255–70.

March J.G. and Simon H.A. (1958). *Organisations*. New York, Wiley.

Margulies N. and Adams J.D. (eds) (1982). *Organisational Development in Health Care Organisations*. Reading, Mass., Addison Wesley.

Miles R. (1966). The affluent organisation. *Harvard Business Review*; May–June, 44: 106–14.

Miller D. and Friesen D.H. (1980). Momentum and revolution in organisation adaptation. *Acad. Manag. Rev*; 591–614.

Miller D. and Friesen P.H. (1984). *Organisations: A Quantum View*. Prentice Hall.

Mintzberg H. (1972) The myth of MIS. California Management Review; Fall: 92–7

Mintzberg H. (1973). *The Nature of Managerial Work*. New York, Harper and Row.

Mintzberg M. (1975). The manager's job: folklore and fact. *Harvard Business Review*.

Mintzberg M. (1979). *The Structuring of Organisations*. Englewood Cliffs, NJ, Prentice Hall.

NHS Management Inquiry (1983). Report, [The Griffiths Report]. London, DHSS.

Nystrom P.C., Hedberg Bo, L.T. and Starbuck W.M. (1976). Interacting processes as organisation designs. In R.H. Kilman, L.R. Pondy and D.P. Stevins (eds), *The Management of Organisation Design*. Vol. 1, 209–30. New York, Elsevier, North Holland.

Nystrom H. (1979). *Creativity and Innovation*. John Wiley and Sons.

Occupational Personality Questionnaire Manual (1984). Esher Green, Surrey, Saville and Holdsworth.

Office of Health Economics (1984). *Understanding the NHS in the 1980s*. Studies of Current Health Problems no. 75, London.

Payne R. (1981). Organisational behaviour. In C.L. Cooper (ed), *Psychology and Management*. London, BPS and MacMillan Press.

Peters T.J. and Waterman R.H. (1982). *In Search of Excellence: Lessons from American's Best-run Companies*. New York, Harper and Row.

Pettigrew A.M. (1973). *Politics of Organisational Decision-Making*. London, Tavistock. [Organisations, People, Society Series, edited by Professor A.B. Cherns.]

Pettigrew A.M. (1985). *The Awakening Giant: Contingency and Change in ICI*. London, Blackwell.

Pettigrew A.M., McKee L and Ferlie E. (1989). Managing strategic service changing in the NHS. *Health Services Management Research*; 2(1): 20–31.

Pfeffer J. (1981). Management as symbolic action: the creation and maintenance of organisational paradigms. In L.L. Cummings and B.N. Shaw (eds), *Research in Organisational Behaviour*. Vol. 3, 1–152, Greenwich, JAI Press.

Pindar K. (1986). The visible persuaders. *Health Care Management*; 1(1): 3–9.

Plant R. (1987). *Managing Change and Making it Stick*. London, Fontana.

Pugh D.S. and Hickson D.J. (1976). *Aston Programme: Volume One*. Saxon House.

Quinn J.B. (1980). *Strategies for Change: Logical Incrementalism*. Homewood, Ill., Irwin.

Rathwell T. (1986). Strategic management – a change agent for the NHS. *Hospital and Health Service Review*; March.

Rickards T. (1985). *Stimulating Innovation: A Systems Approach*. London, Frances Pinter Ltd.

Sayles L.R. (1964). *Management Behaviour*. New York, McGraw-Hill.

Schein E.H. (1984). Coming to a new awareness of organizational culture. *Sloan Management Review*; 25: 5–16.

Schon D.A. (1971). *Beyond the Stable State: Public and Private Learning in a Changing Society*. London, M.T. Smith.

Schwenk C.R. (1988). The cognitive perspective on strategic decision making. *Journal of Management Studies*; 25(1): 41–52.

Silverman D. (1970). *The Theory of Organisations: A Sociological Framework*. London, Heinemann.

Silverman D. and Jones J. (1976). *Organisational Work*. London, MacMillan.

Simon H.A. (1957). *Models of Man*. New York, Wiley.

Smith P. (1987). Appraising your progress as the Unit General Manager. *Hospital and Health Services Review*; November: 256–60.

Solomon E.E. (1986). Private and public sector managers: an empirical investigation of job characteristics and organizational climate. *Journal of Applied Psychology*; 71(2); 247–59.

Sopar H. (1984). A theoretical approach to organizational change. In P.J.D. Drenth. Thierry H., Willems P.J. and de Wolff C.F. *Handbook of Work and Organisational Psychology*, Wiley .

Starbuck W.A. and Hedberg Bo, L.T. (1977). Saving an organisation from a stagnating environment. In H.B. Thorelli (ed), *Structure + Structure = Performance*. Bloomington, Indiana University Press, pp. 249–58.

Stewart R. (1976). *Contrasts in Management*. Maidenhead, McGraw-Hill.

Stewart R. (1982). *Choices for the Manager*. Englewood Cliffs, NJ, Prentice-Hall.

Stewart R. (1985). *The Reality of Management*. Second edition, Heinemann.

Stewart R. (1989). Studies of managerial jobs and behaviour: the ways forward. *Journal of Management Studies*; 26(1): 1–10.

Stewart R. (1989). Pressures and constraints on general management. *Health Services Management Research*; 2(1): 32–37.

Stewart R. and Wyatt S. (1985). Starting from scratch. *Health Service Journal*; September: 1194.

Stinchcombe A.L. (1965). Social structure and organisation. In J.G. March (ed), *Handbook of Organisations*. Chicago, Rand McNally.

Templeton College (1987). Templeton Series on District General Managers. [Stewart R. and others.] Issue Studies Nos. 1–8, Bristol, NHSTA.

Thompson J.D. and Tuden A. (1959). Strategies, structures and processes of organisational decision. In J.D. Thompson *et al*; *Comparative Studies in Administration*. University of Pittsburgh Press.

Tichy N.M. and Beckhard R. (1982). Applied behavioural science for health care organisations. In Margulies and Adams (eds), Organisational development in health care organisations. Reading, Mass., Addison Wesley.

Toulmin S. (1958). *The Uses of Argument.* Cambridge, Cambridge University Press.

Van de Ven A.H. (1980). Problem solving, planning and innovation, Part 1: Test of programme planning method; Part 2: Speculations for theory and practice. *Human Relations Journal;* 33, November–December: 10–11.

Whitley R. (1988). The management sciences and managerial skills. *Organisation Studies;* 9(1): 47–68.

Williams D. and Dopson S. (1988). Managerial relationships in District Health Authorities. *Health Services Management Research;* 1(2): 63–73.

Zaleznik A.(1977). Managers and leaders: are they different? *Harvard Business Review;* May–June: 67–78.

Index

All page references in italics indicate figures and those in bold type represent tables.